Xiang Zhang

Female sex and ER-alpha modulate cardiac ischaemic remodeling

Xiang Zhang

Female sex and ER-alpha modulate cardiac ischaemic remodeling

Cardiomyocyte-specific overexpression of estrogen receptor alpha provides cardioprotection in female mice

Südwestdeutscher Verlag für Hochschulschriften

Impressum / Imprint
Bibliografische Information der Deutschen Nationalbibliothek: Die Deutsche Nationalbibliothek verzeichnet diese Publikation in der Deutschen Nationalbibliografie; detaillierte bibliografische Daten sind im Internet über http://dnb.d-nb.de abrufbar.
Alle in diesem Buch genannten Marken und Produktnamen unterliegen warenzeichen-, marken- oder patentrechtlichem Schutz bzw. sind Warenzeichen oder eingetragene Warenzeichen der jeweiligen Inhaber. Die Wiedergabe von Marken, Produktnamen, Gebrauchsnamen, Handelsnamen, Warenbezeichnungen u.s.w. in diesem Werk berechtigt auch ohne besondere Kennzeichnung nicht zu der Annahme, dass solche Namen im Sinne der Warenzeichen- und Markenschutzgesetzgebung als frei zu betrachten wären und daher von jedermann benutzt werden dürften.

Bibliographic information published by the Deutsche Nationalbibliothek: The Deutsche Nationalbibliothek lists this publication in the Deutsche Nationalbibliografie; detailed bibliographic data are available in the Internet at http://dnb.d-nb.de.
Any brand names and product names mentioned in this book are subject to trademark, brand or patent protection and are trademarks or registered trademarks of their respective holders. The use of brand names, product names, common names, trade names, product descriptions etc. even without a particular marking in this work is in no way to be construed to mean that such names may be regarded as unrestricted in respect of trademark and brand protection legislation and could thus be used by anyone.

Coverbild / Cover image: www.ingimage.com

Verlag / Publisher:
Südwestdeutscher Verlag für Hochschulschriften
ist ein Imprint der / is a trademark of
OmniScriptum GmbH & Co. KG
Heinrich-Böcking-Str. 6-8, 66121 Saarbrücken, Deutschland / Germany
Email: info@svh-verlag.de

Herstellung: siehe letzte Seite /
Printed at: see last page
ISBN: 978-3-8381-5128-1

Zugl. / Approved by: Berlin, Charité Universitätsmedizin, Diss., 2015

Copyright © 2015 OmniScriptum GmbH & Co. KG
Alle Rechte vorbehalten. / All rights reserved. Saarbrücken 2015

Female sex und ER alpha modulate cardiac ischemic remodeling

Dr. med. Xiang Zhang

Contents

1 Abstract/Abstrakt 1
2 Introduction 3
  2.1 Myocardial infarction 3
  2.2 Pathophysiology of myocardial remodeling after myocardial infarction 4
  2.3 Gender perspective 4
  2.4 Effects of E2 and its receptors on cardiovascular system 5
    2.4.1 The effects of E2 on cardiovascular disease 5
    2.4.2 The effects of estrogen receptors on cardiovascular system 7
      2.4.2.1 Estrogen receptor structure and biology 7
      2.4.2.2 Mechanisms of estrogen receptor signaling 8
      2.4.2.3 Role of estrogen receptors in cardiovascular injury 9
        2.4.2.3.1 Cardiovascular effects of ERα in cardiovascular injury 10
  2.6 Cardiomyocyte-specific ERα overexpression mouse model 11
  2.7 Aim of study 13
3 Methodology 14
  3.1 Materials 14
  3.2 Methods 16
    3.2.1 Mouse model of myocardial infarction 16
      3.2.1.1 Transgenic animals 16
      3.2.1.2 Induction of myocardial infarction 16
      3.2.1.3 Organ harvest and preparation of heart section 17
    3.2.2 Cardiac function evaluation with echocardiography 18
    3.2.3 Histology 21
      3.2.3.1 Hematoxylin and eosin staining of paraffin-embedded LV sections 21
      3.2.3.2 Sirius Red staining of paraffin-embedded LV sections 22
        3.2.3.2.1 Sirius Red staining 22
        3.2.3.2.2 Evaluation of collagen deposition in paraffin-embedded LV sections .. 22
      3.2.3.3 Immunofluorescence staining of paraffin-embedded LV sections 23
        3.2.3.3.1 Reagents and antibodies 23
        3.2.3.3.2 Deparaffinization 24
        3.2.3.3.3 Antigen retrieval 24
        3.2.3.3.4 Immunofluorescence staining of paraffin-embedded LV sections 25
        3.2.3.3.5 Quantification of immunoreactivity by pixel intensity 25
    3.2.4 RNA isolation and quantitative real-time polymerase chain reaction 26
      3.2.4.1 RNA isolation and cDNA preparation 27
      3.2.4.2 Quantitative real-time polymerase chain reaction 28
    3.2.5 Protein extraction from myocardial tissue and concentration measurement 30
    3.2.6 Western blot 30
    3.2.7 Statistics 31
4 Results 32
  4.1 ERα overexpression affects echocardiographic parameters at the basal level and after myocardial infarction 32

4.2 ERα enhances cardiac angiogenesis and lymphangiogenesis after myocardial infarction in both sexes 34
4.3 ERα induces the phosphorylation of *JNK* signaling pathway only in female hearts after myocardial infarction 40
4.4 ERα attenuates collagen deposition after myocardial infarction only in female hearts 41
5 Discussion 43
    5.1 Effects of ERα overexpression on the heart 43
    5.2 Effects of ERα overexpression following myocardial infarction 45
        5.2.1 ERα overexpression enhances neovascularization after myocardial infarction 45
        5.2.2 ERα overexpression affects cardiac remodeling following myocardial infarction 49
6 Bibliography 53
Curriculum Vitae I
List of publications III
Acknowledgments/Danksagung IV
List of abbreviations V

1 Abstract/Abstrakt

Experimental studies showed that 17β-estradiol (E2) and activated estrogen receptors (ER) protect the heart from ischemic injury. However, the underlying molecular mechanisms are not well understood. To investigate the role of ER-alpha (ERα) in cardiomyocytes in the setting of myocardial ischemia, we generated transgenic mice with cardiomyocyte-specific overexpression of ERα (ERα-OE) and subjected them to myocardial infarction (MI). At the basal level, female and male ERα-OE mice showed increased left ventricular (LV) mass and LV volume. Two weeks after MI, LV volume was significantly increased and LV wall thickness decreased in female and male WT-mice and male ERα-OE, but not in female ERα-OE mice. ERα-OE enhanced expression of angiogenesis and lymphangiogenesis markers (*VEGF, LYVE-1*), and neovascularization in the peri-infarct area in both sexes. However, an attenuated level of fibrosis and higher phosphorylation of *JNK* signaling pathway could be detected only in female ERα-OE after MI. In conclusion, this study indicates that ERα protects female mouse cardiomyocytes from the sequelae of ischemia through induction of neovascularization in a paracrine fashion and impaired fibrosis, which together may contribute to the attenuation of the adverse consequence of cardiac remodeling.

Abstract

Experimentelle Studien zeigten, dass 17β-Östradiol (E2) und aktivierte Östrogen-Rezeptoren (ER) das Herz vor ischämischen Schäden schützen. Allerdings sind die zugrunde liegenden molekularen Mechanismen nicht gut verstanden. Um die Rolle des ER-alpha (ERα) in Kardiomyozyten während der myokardialen Ischämie zu untersuchen, generierten wir transgene Mäuse mit Kardiomyozyten-spezifischer Überexpression des ERα (ERα-OE) und induzierten einen Myokardinfarkt (MI). Auf Basalniveau zeigten weibliche und männliche ERα-OE-Mäuse im Vergleich zu Wildtyp (WT)-Mäusen eine erhöhte linksventrikuläre (LV) Masse und LV Volumina. Zwei Wochen nach MI waren die LV Volumina deutlich erhöht und die LV Wanddicke in weiblichen und männlichen WT-Mäusen und männlichen ERα-OE verringert, aber nicht in weiblichen ERα-OE Mäusen. ERα-OE verstärkte die Expression von Angiogenese- und Lymphangiogenese-Markern (*VEGF, LYVE-1*) und die Neovaskularisierung im Peri-Infarktbereich bei beiden Geschlechtern. Allerdings konnte nur bei weiblichen ERα-OE-Mäusen ein abgeschwächtes Niveau der Fibrose und eine höhere Aktivierung des *JNK*-Signalweges nach MI festgestellt werden. Zusammenfassend zeigt diese Studie, dass der ERα die weiblichen Kardiomyozyten durch die Induktion der Neovaskularisierung, in parakriner Weise, und verlangsamte Fibrose vor den Folgen der Ischämie schützt, was insgesamt zur besseren Heilung des Myokards nach einem Infarkt führt.

2 Introduction

2.1 Myocardial infarction

The World Health Organization (WHO) estimated that around 17.3 million people annually die due to cardiovascular diseases (CVDs) [1, 2]. By 2030, almost 20.3 million people will die from CVDs each year, mainly from coronary heart disease (CHD, also known as ischemic heart disease, IHD) and stroke [1-3]. Acute myocardial infarction (AMI or MI), more commonly known as a heart attack, which is a common presentation of IHD, occurs when the blood supply to a part of the heart is interrupted, most commonly due to rupture of a vulnerable plaque. The resulting ischemia or oxygen shortage causes damage and potential death of heart tissue. It is a medical emergency and the leading cause of death for both men and women all over the world [4, 5].

MI represents an imbalance between demand and supply of myocardial perfusion which results in ischemia and death of cardiac myocytes [5]. Myocardial ischemia-reperfusion induces an inflammatory response, with damage resulting from both infiltration of circulating inflammatory cells, as well as neutrophil-independent direct actions on myocardium and endothelium [5, 6]. Mechanisms of cell death in MI are complex, including Ca^{2+} overload, ROS generation and impaired mitochondrial regulation [7-9]. In addition, there is incomplete recovery of left ventricular (LV) function. Together, these phenomena contribute to increased risk of ischemic cardiomyopathy, heart failure and death [4, 7, 10].

2.2 Pathophysiology of myocardial remodeling after myocardial infarction

Unfavorable left ventricular remodeling often follows MI. The classical pattern of post-infarction remodeling involves three phases; early compensatory concentric hypertrophy, a subsequent dilative phase leading to eccentric hypertrophy, and the end-stage of progressive wall thinning and dilation [11]. Fibrosis is associated with post infarct remodeling and has important implications for prognosis following MI [12]. In the heart, healing of the damaged area of the LV chamber after MI with a firm fibrous scar is essential for the chamber to continue to pump blood effectively into the tissues. Fibrosis in the infarct and non-infarct zones may become dysregulated and contribute to mixed dilative and hypertrophic remodeling and mixed LV systolic and diastolic dysfunction [13, 14]. Data from clinical studies and animal models suggest that angiogenesis, the formation of new blood vessels, contributes to the preservation of cardiac systolic and diastolic function in myocardial remodeling [15, 16]. Myocardial angiogenesis coupled with a more functional myocardial capillary network may facilitate revascularization and hence preservation of the infarcted myocardium [17].

2.3 Gender perspective

There are considerable epidemiological data showing that pre-menopausal women have a lower incidence and death rate of CVD compared to age-matched men

[18-22]. Additionally, it has been shown that pre-menopausal women have a lower incidence of left ventricular hypertrophy and cardiac remodeling following MI [23, 24]. However, these beneficial effects disappeared rapidly after menopause and the incidence of CVD and its association with mortality reaches a level similar to that of males [25]. This difference has been attributed to the loss of female sex hormone estrogen (17β-estradiol; E2) during the menopausal transition [26-30]. In addition, animal studies support this notion. In most animal studies, females display a lower mortality, less severe hypertrophy, better coronary vasculature adaptations during post-infarction LV remodeling and better perserved cardiac function compared with males [31-33]. Therefore, it has been postulated that female sex hormones, especially E2, may play a cardioprotective role in CVDs and contribute to the mechanistic differences between males and females.

2.4 Effects of E2 and its receptors on cardiovascular system

2.4.1 The effects of E2 on cardiovascular disease

Observational and experimental studies have shown that E2 has protective effects in the myocardium [34-36] and vasculature [37, 38]. Indeed, E2 deficiencies have been associated with an increased risk of mortality after cardiac injury, which was improved by E2 supplementation [39-41]. Experimentally, Hale et al. [35] found that administration of E2 reduced myocardial necrosis and infarct size in rabbits after ischemia and reperfusion (I/R). Kim et al. [42] showed that E2 prevents cardiomyocyte apoptosis through inhibition of reactive oxygen species and differential regulation of p38 kinase isoforms. Additionally, a body of evidence supports that E2 is associated with the improvement of myocardial recovery after I/R injury in different animal models [43-45]. Kolodgie et al. [43] found that an E2-treatment improves contractile function following I/R injury in ovariectomized rats. Jeanes et al. [44] found that protection of the rat heart by E2 after I/R injury is achieved through the reduction of cardiomyocyte death, neutrophil infiltration and oxygen-free radical availability. Squadrito et al. [45] suggested that E2 limits the deleterious intercellular adhesion molecule 1 (ICAM-1) mediated binding of leukocytes to injured myocardium by inhibiting TNF-alpha production and protects against myocardial I/R injury. Furthermore, clinical and animal studies have also shown that E2 may modulate cardiac hypertrophy [34, 46-49]. For example, van Eickels et al. [34] and Patten et al. [49] have demonstrated that long-term E2 treatment attenuated the hypertrophic response to pressure overload in ovariectomized mice. Furthermore, E2 has often been shown to prevent vascular dysfunction and injury. E2 accelerates endothelial recovery and increases nitric oxide (NO) production after de-endothelializing balloon injury [50]. These data support the hypothesis that E2 may contribute to the sexual dimorphism in the heart and to a better outcome of cardiovascular system (CVS). However, the mechanisms by which E2 leads to cardioprotection are not completely understood.

2.4.2 The effects of estrogen receptors on cardiovascular system

It has been shown that E2 exerts its beneficial effects via binding to estrogen receptors (ERs) [51]. The two distinctive ERs best known to date are the original estrogen receptor-alpha (ERα) [52, 53] and the more recently discovered estrogen receptor-beta (ERβ) [54, 55]. They are encoded by distinct genes with different levels of expression in various tissue types [56]. Both ERs are expressed and localized in different cardiac cell types of humans and rodents, such as cardiomyocytes, fibroblasts and endothelial cells [57-63].

2.4.2.1 Estrogen receptor structure and biology

Both ERs belong to the nuclear receptor superfamily [64]. Upon binding of E2, these receptors translocate into the nucleus, where they act as transcription factors regulating gene expression of E2-target genes [64]. ERs contain 6 regions in their protein structure, namely: A, B, C, D, E and F which form functionally different but interacting domains (Figure 1).

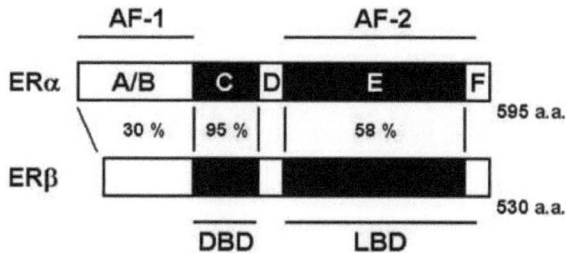

Figure 1. Schematic representation of domain organizations of human ERα and ERβ with percentages indicating homology between the two receptors. Taken from [65].

Although ERα and ERβ are encoded separately, they share a high degree of homology. The A/B region located in the N-terminus of the protein encompasses the activation function (AF)-1 domain responsible for ligand-independent transactivation [64, 65]. The AF-1 domain is the least conserved part among the two ERs with 30% homology. The most conserved domain among ERs is the DNA-binding domain (DBD) corresponding to the C region, with 95% homology between ERα and ERβ subtypes. The DBD is responsible for binding to estrogen response elements (EREs) within the promoter of target gene [64, 65]. The hinge region localized in the D domain contains the nuclear localization signal. The C-terminus of the protein contains the ligand-dependent transactivation domain AF-2, the ligand binding domain (LBD) and the homo-/heterodimerization site [64, 65]. Homology between the E/F regions of both proteins is only 58%, explaining differences in ligand-binding affinities between the two receptors [64, 65].

2.4.2.2 Mechanisms of estrogen receptor signaling

ERs act by regulating gene expression in two modes, including a genomic and a non-genomic pathway [51]. The "genomic" signaling mode involves binding of ERs with specific DNA sequences called EREs which are located within regulatory regions of target genes [51]. However, ERs can also regulate gene expression without directly binding to DNA. This occurs through protein-protein interactions with other DNA-binding transcription factors in the nucleus [51]. In addition to genomic action, the second mode of action is the rapid "non-genomic" action of E2. It is mediated by membrane ERs activating several pathways, including: phosphatidyl inositol 3 kinase/protein kinase B (PI3K/AKT), cAMP/protein kinase A (PKA), phospholipase C (PLC)/protein kinase C (PKC) and mitogen-activated protein kinases (MAPK) signaling pathway [51, 65].

2.4.2.3 Role of estrogen receptors in cardiovascular injury

ER signaling in CVS is complex. In order to understand the role of ERs in CVS, genetic mouse models and pharmacologic studies were used [66, 67]. Zhai et al. [68] and Wang et al. [69] demonstrated that ERα is associated with less severe cardiac damage and lower incidence of arrhythmias following I/R injury using female ERα-knockout (ERKO) mice. Babiker et al. [70] showed that E2 treatment did result in smaller infarct sizes in ovariectomized female ERKO mice, but increased the infarct size in ovariectomized ERβ-knockout (BERKO) mice. Conversely, Booth et al. [71] reported that acute treatment with an ERα selective agonist, propyl-pyrazole-triol (PPT) resulted in significant reduction of infarct size in rabbit hearts of I/R injury. In another study, treatment with an ERβ-selective agonist, diarylpropionitrile (DPN) can increase functional recovery in ovariectomized female mice after I/R injury [72]. Altogether, these studies indicate that probably either ERα or ERβ or both could have beneficial effects during cardiovascular injury, and these studies did not provide a clear answer as to which ER mediates the effects of E2 in CVS. In this study, we focused on the role of ERα in CVS under stress.

2.4.2.3.1 Cardiovascular effects of ERα in cardiovascular injury

ERα is one of the known ERs which mediates, at least partly, the beneficial effects of E2 on the heart during stress, in a genomic or non-genomic manner [51]. In clinical studies, increased expression of ERα have been detected in the heart of patients with aortic stenosis and dilated cardiomyopathy, most likely as a compensatory mechanism [60, 62]. The absence of ERα is associated with an increased presence of atherosclerotic plaque in humans, especially in premenopausal women [73, 74]. Consistent with these clinical findings, animal studies have demonstrated that ERKO mouse hearts subjected to I/R had fewer viable cardiomyocytes, decreased coronary flow rate, marked myocardial edema, more prominent mitochondrial damage, and decreased functional recovery of contractility and compliance compared with wild type (WT)-mice [68, 69]. By contrast, Novotny et al. [75] demonstrated that in aged ovariectomized female rats, acute in vivo administration of an ERα-selective agonists, PPT was able to reduce infarct size and ischemic injury. Jeanes et al. [44] found that administration of an ERα-selective agonists, ERA-45 following phenomenon of I/R injury resulted in the reduction of cardiomyocyte death, neutrophil infiltration and oxygen-free radical availability on ovariectomized female rats. Vornehm et al. [76] found that post-ischemic administration of the ERα agonist PPT significantly increases myocardial vascular endothelial growth factor receptor (VEGF) production in rat hearts using Langendorff perfusion system. Considering the protective effects of VEGF on the heart, it has been postulated that this ERα agonist may mediate cardiac protection through increased VEGF expression. Indeed, a recent study [77] reveals that E2 regulates the angiogenesis via ERα after MI. In the heart, E2 acts mainly via ERα to enhance the VEGF transcription, the capillary density, and the development of coronary microvasculature [77].

Taken together, these findings indicate that E2-induced cardiovascular effects are, at least partly, mediated by ERα under stress, and it is of critical importance to understand the relative role of this receptor in the heart.

2.6 Cardiomyocyte-specific ERα overexpression mouse model

The activity of ERα is tightly regulated in a cell specific manner through complex processes which are still not fully understood. Since cardiomyocytes have greater vulnerability to ischemia compared with other cell types and their survival determines the outcome after MI [78], we aimed to analyze the specific role of ERα in cardiomyocytes during ischemia. We therefore generated a transgenic mouse model with a cardiomyocyte-specific ERα overexpression (ERα-OE, in collaboration with Dr. F. Jaisser, INSERM, Paris) and subjected mice of both sexes to MI.

This transgenic mouse model with cardiomyocyte-specific ERα-OE was generated using the tet-off system. Briefly, the previously described tetO-ERα mouse strain [79] carrying a transgene composed of a coding sequence for murine ERα placed under the regulatory control of a tet-operator promoter (tet-op-ERα mice) (kindly provided by PA Furth, University of Maryland, Baltimore, USA) was crossed with the previously described α-MHCtTA transactivator mouse strain [80] (kindly provided by GI Fishman, Columbia University, NY). This allows to obtain MHCtTA/tetO-ERα double transgenic (ERα-OE) mice with conditional, cardiomyocyte-specific ERα expression (Figure 2).

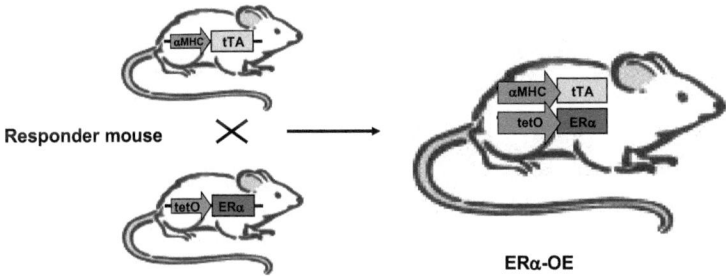

Figure 2. Inducible double transgenic mice with cardiomyocyte-specific ERα overexpression (ERα-OE) were generated through mating of transgenic ERα (tetO-ERα) and transgenic α-MHC-tTA mice using tet-Off system.

2.7 Aim of study

E2 exerts its beneficial effects on the myocardium during stress via ER. During and after MI, administration of ERα-selective agonist has protective effects in the heart. By contrast, ERKO animals have a poorer outcome after MI. We therefore hypothesized that ERα contributes to the myocardial protection after cardiac injury, and this differs in male and female. To test this hypothesis, we used a transgenic mouse model with a cardiomyocyte-specific ERα overexpression (ERα-OE) and subjected mice of both sexes to MI. This model was designed to address the following questions:

1. has ERα beneficial effects on the heart under stress.

2. may ERα contribute to the sexual dimorphism in the heart and to a better cardiac outcome after MI.

3. does ERα contribute to the attenuation of cardiac remodeling after MI?

3 Methodology

3.1 Materials

Materials used in this study show in table 1-5

Table 1. Various devices

Various devices	Company, Country
Centrifuge 5417R	Eppendorf, Germany
Light microscope	Carl Zeiss, Germany
Fluorescent microscope	Olympus, Japan
Fluorescent microscope	Leica, Germany
Real-Time PCR System	Applied Biosystems 7300 Foster USA
Master cycler gradient	Applied Biosystems, USA
Thermo mixer Compact	Eppendorf, Germany
PH-Meter	Five easy, USA
Echocardiography-Vevo 770	Toronto Ontario, Canada
Microm cool-cut	Microm, Germany
Pressure cooker	Silit, Germany
Blotting apparatus	Bio Rad, Germany

Table 2. Surgical material

Surgical material	Company, Country
Fine Dissecting Scissors (310-404)	Heiland, Germany
anatomical forceps straight (310-173)	Heiland, Germany
curved anatomical forceps eye (310-176)	Heiland, Germany
Micro scissors (no. 91500-09)	FST, Germany
Eye needle holder (310-196)	Heiland, Germany
micro needle holders (no. 12061-01)	FST, Germany
Hemostat	Heiland, Germany
Polypropylene thread 7-0	Ethicon, Prolene
Silk thread 6-0	Spule, Fa. Ernst, Germany
stereo zoom microscope	Leica MZ125, Germany
fiber optic light source	KL1500 LCD SCHOTT, Germany
HA Mini Vent ventilator for mice	Harvard Apparatus, USA
Depilatory cream	Elca Med, Germany
heating pad	Hans Dinslage GmbH, Germany
IV catheter	BD, Ireland

Methodology

Table 3. Chemical reagents

Chemical reagents	Company, Country
Ethanol 100%	Merck KGaA, Germany
Isopropanol	Merck KGaA, Germany
Trizol	Invitrogen, Karlsruhe, Germany
Ultra–pure water	Biochrom GmbH, Germany
DEPC	Carl Roth GmbH, Germany
EDTA	Carl Roth GmbH, Germany
NaOH	Merck KGaA, Germany
NaCl	Carl Roth GmbH, Germany
Tris	Carl Roth GmbH, Germany
Glycine	Carl Roth GmbH, Germany
SDS	Carl Roth GmbH, Germany
TEMED	Carl Roth GmbH, Germany
Brilliant blue 250	Carl Roth GmbH, Germany
Ponceau S solution	Sigma, Germany
Triton X-100	Carl Roth GmbH, Germany

Table 4. Staining solutions

Staining solutions	Company, Country
Hematoxylin	Sigma, Germany
Eosin	Sigma, Germany
Sirius Red	Fluka, Germany
DAPI	Dako, USA
Acetic acid	Carl Roth GmbH, Germany
Bovine serum albumin (BSA)	Sigma, Germany
xylene	Merck KGaA, Germany
Citric acid	Carl Roth GmbH, Germany
35% BSA	Sigma Aldrich, USA
PBS tablets	CalBiochem, Germany
Vectashield H-100	Vector laboratories, CA

Table 5. Nucleic acids analysis

Nucleic acids analysis	Company, Country
10 × RT buffer	Applied biosystems, USA
dNTPs	Applied biosystems, USA
10 × RT random primers	Applied biosystems, USA
RNase inhibitor	Applied biosystems, USA
multiScribe Reverse Transcriptase	Applied biosystems, USA
Fast SYBR Green Power mastermix	Applied biosystems, USA
96-well Multiply PCR plate	Applied biosystems, USA

3.2 Methods

3.2.1 Mouse model of myocardial infarction

3.2.1.1 Transgenic animals

Inducible double transgenic mice with ERα-OE were generated through mating of monotransgenic ERα (tetO-mERα) and monotransgenic α-MHC-tTA mice using tet-Off system (for more details, see introduction capital). Since cardiac phenotype and function of monotransgenic tetO-mERα and α-MHC-tTA mice did not significantly differ from wild type-littermates (WT), we did not include the monotransgenic mice in further analysis, and only the WT were used as control. All animal experiments were approved by and conducted in accordance with the guidelines set out by the State Agency for Health and Social Affairs (LaGeSo, Berlin, Germany, G 0360/08).

3.2.1.2 Induction of myocardial infarction

Mice were anesthetized with a mixture of ketamine (2.5 ml/kg) and xylazine (0.8 ml/kg) by intraperitoneal injection, incubated and ventilated with a small-animal ventilator (Starling Ideal Ventilator, Harvard Apparatus USA) with room air at a respiratory rate of 220 breaths per minute with a ventilatory tidal volume of 0.2 ml [81].

Before doing operation, loss of pedal reflex was used as an index of onset of the surgical anesthesia. After successful intubation, the mouse was fixed with hind limbs on the right side of the body. Using a heater, the body temperature was kept at 37°C.

At first, the mouse was shaved on the left side of chest, and these areas were cleaned and sterilized with polyvidone-iodine. To perform a thoracotomy at the left side, the mouse was relocated on its right side. The skin was incised and the subcutaneous tissue was dissected, then a left thoracotomy was performed via the 4th intercostal space and the lungs retracted to expose the heart [82]. After opening the pericardium, the left anterior descending coronary artery (LAD) was ligated with a 7.0 polypropylene suture near its origin between the pulmonary outflow tract and the edge of the atrium. Ligation deemed successful when the anterior wall of the left ventricle turned pale [82-84]. The lungs were inflated by increasing positive end-expiratory pressure. Thorax, the muscle layer and skin were closed separately with a 6.0 silk suture [82, 83]. Mice were kept on a heating pad until they recovered. Sham group of mice underwent the similar surgical procedure without tightening the suture around the coronary artery.

3.2.1.3 Organ harvest and preparation of heart section

The heart tissues were harvested 14 days after MI. The Mice were anesthetized with isoflurane and killed by cervical dislocation. The chest was opened with scissors and the heart was removed quickly. Thereafter, the heart was washed free of blood in a buffer solution (PBS) and subsequently weighed. The left ventricle was separated from the atria and the right ventricle. Then the isolated left ventricle was also weighed and dissected for further processing in the following three parts: part 1 apex, part 2 middle part (infarct and infarct border zone), and part 3 remote area. Part 1 and 3 were frozen for mRNA determination in liquid nitrogen at −196°C, Part 2 for histological examination was fixed immediately in formalin.

To determine the ratio of heart weight / tibia length (HW/TL), tibia was dissected and its length was determined using a caliper.

3.2.2 Cardiac function evaluation with echocardiography

Echocardiography is a diagnostic test that uses ultrasound waves to create an image of the heart muscle. Ultrasound waves that rebound or echo off the heart can visualize the heart and quantify cardiac function [84, 85]. Ultrasound waves are differentially transmitted through the various soft tissues, relative to their acoustic impedance and density. At the border of two tissues with different acoustic impedances an acoustic impedance mismatch occurs and some of the sound waves are reflected and returned to the transducer. The signal from reflected ultrasound waves is transformed into electrical currents, processed and an image is created and displayed [84, 85].

Echocardiography was performed 1 day before surgery and 14 days after MI. Mice were first anesthetized with oxygen containing 3ppm isoflurane, during echocardiography with oxygen containing 1.5ppm isoflurane. Mice were placed on a heated platform in supine position with all legs taped to ECG electrodes for heart rate monitoring and the chest was shaved and depilated. Cardiac function was assessed by ultrasound using an echocardiography system (Vevo 770 High-Resolution Imaging System, Toronto, Canada) equipped with a 20-55 MHz transducer. All data were transferred to a computer for offline analysis.

Conventional echocardiographic measurements were obtained from B mode images acquired from the parasternal long-axis view. As shown in Figure 3A-3C, the volume of the LV endocardium volume in systole and diastole (LVVol, s; LVVol, d) and LV mass were measured from 2-dimensional parasternal long-axis views. LVVol, s and LVVol, d, LV mass were calculated according to the following formula [86, 87]:

$$LVVol, s = \frac{4\pi}{3} \times \frac{LV\ axis\ (s)}{2} \times \left(\frac{LV\ area\ (s)}{\pi \left(\frac{LV\ axis\ (s)}{2} \right)} \right)^2$$

$$LVVol, d = \frac{4\pi}{3} \times \frac{LV\ axis\ (d)}{2} \times \left(\frac{LV\ area\ (d)}{\pi \left(\frac{LV\ axis\ (d)}{2} \right)} \right)^2$$

$$LVM = 1,05 \times \left[\left(\frac{5}{6} \times epicardial\ area\ (d) \times (epicardial\ axis\ (d) + T) \right) - \left(\frac{5}{6} \times endocardial\ area\ (d) \times endocardial\ axis\ (d) \right) \right]$$

$$T = \sqrt{\frac{epicardial\ area\ (d)}{\pi}} - \sqrt{\frac{endocardial\ area\ (d)}{\pi}}$$

Methodology

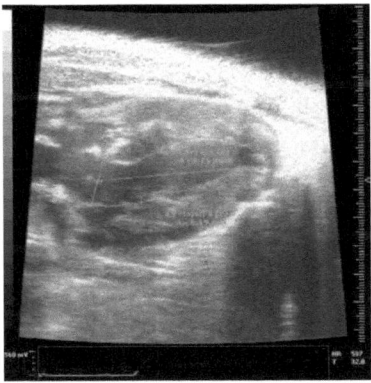

Figure 3 A. Vevo Ultrasound Imaging System. The volume of the LV endocardium volume in systole (LVVol, s) was measured from B-mode ultrasound image of a parasternal long-axis view of a mouse left ventricle.

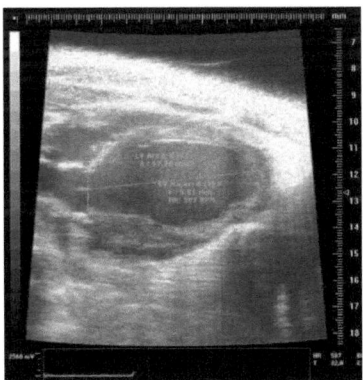

Figure 3 B. Vevo Ultrasound Imaging System. The volume of the LV endocardium volume in diastole (LVVol, d) was measured from B-mode ultrasound image of a parasternal long-axis view of a mouse left ventricle.

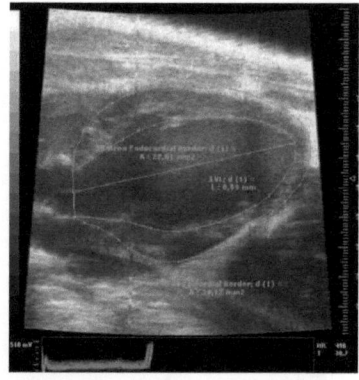

Figure 3 C. Vevo Ultrasound Imaging System. LV mass was measured from B-mode ultrasound image of a parasternal long-axis view of a mouse left ventricle.

3.2.3 Histology

3.2.3.1 Hematoxylin and eosin staining of paraffin-embedded LV sections

The 3-μm paraffin-embedded LV sections were placed at 60°C for 1 h, incubated in xylene 2 times at RT for 10 min and then transferred sequentially into 100% Ethanol (EtOH), 96% EtOH, 85% EtOH, and 70% EtOH for 5 min at RT. Sections were rinsed in deionized water for 5 min. After being deparaffinized, all sections were treated with hematoxylin for 20 min, with distilled water for 3 min and treated with 0.1% eosin for 3 min. After being transferred sequentially into 70% EtOH, 96% EtOH, 100% EtOH, and 100% EtOH for 2min at RT, all sections were transferred into xylene for 3 min at RT. Finally sections were mounted with vectamount mounting medium and visualized by light microscopy.

3.2.3.2 Sirius Red staining of paraffin-embedded LV sections

3.2.3.2.1 Sirius Red staining

The 3-μm paraffin-embedded LV sections were placed at 60°C for 1 h, incubated twice in xylene at RT for 5 min and then transferred sequentially into 100% EtOH, 96% EtOH, 80% EtOH, and 50% EtOH for 20 s at RT. Sections were rinsed in deionized water for 1 min. After being deparaffinized, all sections were treated with 0.1% Sirius Red solution for 30 min, rinsed with 0.1% acetic acid for 5 min and rinsed with distilled water for 20 s, and then transferred sequentially into 50% EtOH, 80% EtOH, 96% EtOH, and 100% EtOH for 20 s at RT. Finally, sections were mounted with vectamount mounting medium and visualized by motorized upright microscope (Olympus BX61).

3.2.3.2.2 Evaluation of collagen deposition in paraffin-embedded LV sections

To analyze the changes in fibrotic areas, microscopic images of collagen deposition were quantified using Media Cybernetics Image Pro PLUS software (Bethesda, MD). A threshold was used to select pixels occupied by collagens, as represented by Sirius Red staining, and the image was binarized by setting these collagen regions to white (pixel value, 255) and background pixels to black (pixel value, 0) to form a "mask" of Sirius Red staining. Firstly choosing irregular area of interest (AOI) to define measuring area, then using Image Pro's Count/Size tool, objects with a pixel intensity of 255 were counted in each section. The area was automatically measured using Image Pro's calibrated area measurement tool. The percentage of fibrosis area to entire cross-sectional area of LV was calculated.

3.2.3.3 Immunofluorescence staining of paraffin-embedded LV sections

3.2.3.3.1 Reagents and antibodies

The blood and lymphatic capillaries are histologically very similar in appearance, and it has been very difficult to distinguish lymphatic capillaries from blood capillaries without electron microscopic examination. However, recently it has become possible to distinguish lymphatic and blood vessels from each other by using antibodies against *CD31* (*PECAM-1*, platelet endothelial cell adhesion molecule-1) and *LYVE-1* (Lymphatic vessel endothelial hyaluronan receptor-1) [88, 89]. Details of the primary antibodies and secondary antibodies used for this study are given in table 6 and 7.

Table 6. Primary antibodies

Primary antibody	Dilution	Source	Code number	Incubation
CD31	1/200	Santa Cruz	(M-20)sc-1056-R	Over night
LYVE-1	1/50	Santa Cruz	(Xb-13)sc-80170	Over night

Table 7. Secondary antibodies

Secondary antibody	Dilution	Source	Code number	Incubation
FITC goat anti-rabbit	1/100	Jackson Lab.	111-075-045	1 h
Cy3 rabbit anti-rat	1/100	Jackson Lab.	312-165-003	30 min

3.2.3.3.2 Deparaffinization

The 3-µm paraffin-embedded LV sections were placed at 60°C for 1 h, incubated in xylene 2 times at RT for 5 min, and then transferred sequentially into 100% EtOH, 95% EtOH, 70% EtOH, and 50% EtOH for 5 min at RT. Sections were rinsed in deionized water for 5 min and stored in PBS.

3.2.3.3.3 Antigen retrieval

To determine the optimal condition for antigen retrieval, two different epitope retrieval methods were used. 1). For heat induced epitope retrieval in a pressure cooker sections were heated in citrate buffer, 10 mM, pH 6, for 5 min followed by a slow cooling for 20 min. 2). For heat induced epitope retrieval in a microwave slides were incubated thrice at 800 W for 5 min in citrate buffer, 10 mM, pH 6 followed by a slow cooling for 20 min. As presented in table 8, after pre-test, we only found positive signals using antibodies against *CD31 and LYVE-1* for heat induced epitope retrieval in a pressure cooker.

Table 8. Epitope retrieval methods

Antibody	Microwave *	Boiling **	Clone
CD31	-	+	(M-20)sc-1506-R
LYVE-1	-	+	(Xb-13)sc-80170

* 5 min at 800 W in citrate buffer, pH 6, thrice

** 5 min in a pressure cooker in citrate buffer, pH 6.

3.2.3.3.4 Immunofluorescence staining of paraffin-embedded LV sections

All slides were rinsed in TBS thrice before blocking with 1% BSA-PBS for 1 h. Tissues were outlined with a liquid Blocker Super Pap Pen to minimize the volume (20–30 ul) of antibody solution needed for staining. Several antibodies were used: 1:200 dilution of *CD31*; 1:50 dilution of *LYVE-1*. Antibodies were diluted in PBS containing 0.1% BSA and added to each tissue section and incubated over night at 4 °C in a humidified chamber. The sections were rinsed thrice with PBS, incubated with a fluorescent dye conjugated secondary antibody (*Cy3* rabbit anti-rat, *FITC* goat anti-rabbit, Jackson USA, respectively) diluted in PBS with 0.1% BSA for 1 h. Slides were rinsed thrice in PBS and Nuclei were stained with 6-diamidino-2-phenylindole (DAPI). Finally sections were mounted with Vectashield H-100 and viewed on a motorized upright fluorescence microscope (Olympus BX61). Negative controls included sections in which either the primary antibodies, secondary antibodies or both were omitted.

3.2.3.3.5 Quantification of immunoreactivity by pixel intensity

Microscopic images of blood vasculature and lymphatic vessel were quantified using Media Cybernetics Image Pro PLUS software. A threshold was used to select pixels occupied by blood vessels, as represented by *CD31* staining, and the image was binarized by setting these blood vessel regions to white (pixel value, 255) and background pixels to black (pixel value, 0) to form a "mask" of positive *CD31* staining. Firstly choosing irregular AOI to define measuring area, then using Image Pro's Count/Size tool, objects with a pixel intensity of 255 (i.e., *CD31*-positive) were counted in each section. The area was automatically measured using Image Pro's calibrated area measurement tool. The ratio of area of *CD31* expressing vessels to whole LV cross-sectional area was calculated. A similar method was used to evaluate *LYVE-1* expressing vessels.

3.2.4 RNA isolation and quantitative real-time polymerase chain reaction

Quantitative polymerase chain reaction (qPCR), also called real-time polymerase chain reaction, is a common laboratory technique of molecular biology based on the polymerase chain reaction (PCR), which is used to amplify and simultaneously quantify a targeted DNA molecule [90]. The quantity can be either an absolute number of copies or a relative amount when normalized to DNA input or additional normalizing genes. Real-time qPCR involves the use of a fluorescent reporter molecule to monitor the progress of the amplification reaction. Fluorescence is measured at each amplification cycle; it increases step-wise and is proportional to the amplicon concentration. The greater the amount of initial DNA template in the sample, the lower is the number of cycles necessary to reach fluorescence threshold (Ct value). In this study, reaction mixture containing SYBR green fluorescent was used and relative gene expression was calculated using

-ΔΔCt method [90].

3.2.4.1 RNA isolation and cDNA preparation

Mouse heart RNA was prepared using Trizol reagent according to the manufacturer's protocol. Heart samples were frozen at -80°C until usage. 1 ml of RNA-Bee was added to 100 mg of myocardium for mechanical homogenization for 20 s using Fast Prep apparatus FP120 (Thermo Fisher Scientific). Following a second homogenization by shaking for 30 min at 4°C, 200 µl of chloroform were added. After vortexing, the sample was centrifuged at 14000 U/min for 10 min at 4°C and the upper transparent phase containing RNA was carefully taken. RNA was precipitated with isopropanol over night at -20°C and centrifuged for 30 min at 14000 U/min at 4°C. The RNA containing pellet was washed with 80% ethanol and centrifuged for 5 min at 8000 U/min at 4°C. The resulting RNA pellet was dissolved in sterile, DEPC-treated water. RNA concentration was measured, aliquoted and stored at - 80°C until usage.

0.5µg of pure high quality RNA was transcribed into cDNA using SuperScript™ II reverse transcriptase with random primers according to the protocol provided by the manufacturer in a total volume of 20 ul (table 9).

Table 9. Reverse transcription-cDNA synthesis

Reagent	Volume (µl)
0.5µg RNA	4
10 x random primers	2
dNTPs (100mM)	0.8
Superscript II RT enzyme	1
10 x buffer	2
RNase inhibitor (40 u/ul)	0.25
DEPC-H_2O	9.95
Total volume	20

3.2.4.2 Quantitative real-time polymerase chain reaction

Quantification of expression levels of the mouse *VEGF and LYVE-1* were performed by real time PCR using SYBRGreen. The housekeeping gene Hypoxanthine Phosphoribosyltransferase (*HPRT*) was used to normalize the results. Results were analyzed using the Applied Biosystems 7300 Real-Time PCR software. Real-time PCR was carried out for 40 cycles (95°C 15 s, 60°C 1 min, table 10 and 11). Primer sequences used for amplification are listed in (table 12).

Table 10. Real-time PCR reaction mixture

Reagent	Volume (µl)
SYBR Green II mastermix	10
Forward primer	3
Reverse primer	1
Ultra-pure water	1
cDNA	5
Final volume/reaction	20

Table 11. Thermal Cycler profile

Stage	Repetitions	Temperature	Time
1	1	95.0 °C	10 min
2	40	95.0 °C	15 s
		60.0 °C	1 min
3 (Dissociation)	1	95.0 °C	15 s
		60.0 °C	1 min
		95.0 °C	15 s
		60.0 °C	15 s

All primers used in this study show in table 12

Table 12. Primers for qRT-PCR

Gene	Size (bp)	Sequence
m-VEGF α	94	FW: 5-GCA GCT TGA GTT AAA CGA ACG-3
		FW: 5-GGT TCC CGA AAC CCT GAG-3
m-LYVE-1	91	FW: 5-GAA GCA GCT GGG TTT GGA-3
		RV: 5-CGT AGC AAA CAG CCA GCA C-3
m-HPRT	78	FW:5-CACAGGACTAGAACACCTGC-3
		RV: 5-GCTGGTGAAAAGGACCTCT-3

Table 12. List of all primers for quantitative Real-Time polymerase Chain Reaction: the RT-qPCR was performed with gene-specific, intron-spanning primers. The annealing temperature was 60°C.

3.2.5 Protein extraction from myocardial tissue and concentration measurement

First, the weight of tissue samples was determined. Lysis buffer was added to frozen samples and homogenized using Fast Prep apparatus FP120 (Thermo Fisher Scientific). After homogenization, 10% SDS was added, and the samples were mixed briefly and incubated for 20 min on ice. Subsequently, the samples were centrifuged for 10 min at 14000 U/min. The aqueous supernatant was transferred into a new tube and stored at -80°C.

To determine the protein concentration, 20 µl of a 1:40 dilution of isolated protein samples was added into 300 µl dye mixture (Pierce™ BCA Protein Assay, mixing 50 parts of BCA Reagent A with 1 part of BCA Reagent B) and incubated for 30 min at 37°C. The protein was measured in a 96-well plate with flat bottom using ELISA plate reader at $\lambda=550$ nm. As reference, dilution series of albumin were used.

3.2.6 Western blot

Western blot analyses were performed using whole LV tissues isolated from female and male ERα-OE mice (n≥8) or WT-mice (n≥8). Briefly, for each sample, 25µg of protein was loaded into a 10% polyacrylamide gel, electrophoresed, and transferred to a nitrocellulose membrane. Western blot analyses were performed using a standard protocol with specific primary antibodies against mitogen-activated protein kinase c-jun N-terminal kinase *JNK1/3* (C-17, Santa Cruz, dilution 1:200), *p-JNK* (G-7, Santa Cruz, dilution 1:200). Specific bands were visualized using ECL™ detection kit (GE Healthcare) and band density was analyzed with Image J software (NIH).

3.2.7 Statistics

All data are presented as mean ± standard error of the means (SEM). Statistical analysis was performed using One-way ANOVA followed by Bonferroni's test to compare multiple groups, and two-tailed Student's t-test to compare the mean of two groups. Statistical analyses were performed using Graphpad Prism 5.01 software. Differences with $p \leq 0.05$ were considered significant.

4 Results

4.1 ERα overexpression affects echocardiographic parameters at the basal level and after myocardial infarction

The left ventricular mass (LVM), ratio of LVM to tibia length (LVM/TL), left ventricular wall thickness (LVW), left ventricular diastolic and systolic volume (LVVol, d and LVVol, s) were measured and compared between sexes and genotypes and among all treatment groups in the current work.

As shown in table 13, at the basal level, LVM, LVM/TL, LVVol,d and LVVol,s were significantly elevated in both female and male ERα-OE mice hearts, compared to their respective WT mice (LVM, female: 103.66±3.22 vs. 84.69±2.97; male: 134.98±5.91 vs. 113.97±2.10, $p<0.05$. LVM/TL, female: 6.23±0.20 vs. 5.19±0.17; male: 7.98±0.34 vs. 6.76±0.13, $p<0.05$. LVVol, d, female: 59.75±3.25 vs. 40.90±1.81; male 63.56±3.52 vs. 52.71±2.14, $p<0.05$. LVVol, s, female: 31.23±3.24 vs. 14.01±1.26; male 31.63±2.93 vs. 19.98±1.18, $p<0.05$), indicating that cardiomyocyte-specific ERα-OE leads to a spontaneous development of eccentric cardiac hypertrophy in both sexes. This was due to in both sexes an increase in ventricular diastolic and systolic volumes, but not wall thickness. After MI, neither female nor male in ERα-OE and WT mice showed any significant changes of LVM/TL. Just as female and male WT mice, male ERα-OE mice showed significant increases in LV volumes (LVVol, d, WT-female: 67.43±6.14 vs.

40.90±1.81; WT-male: 95.77±8.95 vs. 52.71±2.14, p<0.05; ERα-OE-male, 94.53±5.32 vs. 63.56±3.52, p<0.05. LVVol, s, WT-female: 47.51±6.64 vs. 14.01±1.26; WT-male: 67.74±10.72 vs. 19.98±1.18, p<0.05; ERα-OE-male, 69.40±5.55 vs. 31.63±2.93, p<0.05) and decreases in LVW (WT-female: 0.57±0.01 vs. 0.63±0.02; WT-male: 0.62±0.01 vs. 0.71±0.01, p<0.05; ERα-OE-male, 0.65±0.02 vs. 0.73±0.01, p<0.05) two weeks after MI. In contrast, female ERα-OE showed no significant changes either in parameters of LV dilatation or wall thickness.

Table 13. Morphological parameters and echocardiographic parameters

Genotype	WT-mice				ERα-OE mice			
Sex	Female		Male		Female		Male	
Treatment	sham (n=12)	MI (n=11)	sham (n=18)	MI (n=12)	sham (n=14)	MI (n=9)	sham (n=15)	MI (n=9)
BW [g]	22.03 ±0.52	21.48 ±0.54	28.17 ±0.60	28.58 ±0.78	22.33 ±0.52	21.31 ±0.53	27.64 ±0.57	27.53 ±0.75
TL [mm]	16.32 ±0.13	16.35 ±0.16	16.86 ±0.09	16.81 ±0.16	16.66 ±0.11	16.39 ±0.13	16.91 ±0.10	16.54 ±0.16
LVM [mg]	84.69 ±2.97	90.94 ±1.99	113.97 ±2.10	121.10 ±4.31	103.66§ ±3.22	105.93 ±4.07	134.98§ ±5.91	130.90 ±4.27
LVM/TL [mg/mm]	5.19 ±0.17	5.57 ±0.14	6.76 ±0.13	7.20 ±0.24	6.23§ ±0.20	6.46 ±0.24	7.98§ ±0.34	7.90 ±0.23
LVW [mm]	0.63 ±0.02	0.57* ±0.01	0.71 ±0.01	0.62* ±0.01	0.64 ±0.01	0.62 ±0.02	0.73 ±0.01	0.65* ±0.02
LVVol,d [µl]	40.90 ±1.81	67.43* ±6.14	52.71 ±2.14	95.77* ±8.95	59.75§ ±3.25	74.64 ±4.76	63.56§ ±3.52	94.53* ±5.32
LVVol,s [µl]	14.01 ±1.26	47.51* ±6.64	19.98 ±1.18	67.74* ±10.72	31.23§ ±3.24	50.50 ±6.30	31.63§ ±2.93	69.40* ±5.55

Table 13. Morphological and echocardiographic parameters 2 weeks after sham and MI surgery in female and male WT- and ERα-OE mice. Data are means ±SEM. MI: Myocardial Infarction; Sham: sham operation; F: female; M: male; n: Number of animals; BW: Body weight; TL: Tibia length; HW: heart weight; LVM: left ventricular mass; LVW: left ventricular wall thickness; LVVol, d: left ventricular diastolic volume; LVVol, s: left ventricular systolic volume. All data are shown as Mean ± SEM. *p<0.05 MI vs. sham, §p<0.05 ERα-OE vs. WT.

To summarize, ERα-OE leads to the spontaneous development of eccentric type of cardiac hypertrophy in both sexes. MI induces pathological changes in cardiac morphology changes after MI in all groups except in female ERα-OE mice. This suggests an improved myocardial adaptation after myocardial infarction in female ERα-OE.

4.2 ERα enhances cardiac angiogenesis and lymphangiogenesis after myocardial infarction in both sexes

In H&E-Staining of paraffin-embedded heart sections of ERα-OE mice, we observed increased occurrence of vascular-like structures in the peri-infarct area, which were found to a lesser extent in the WT mice (Figure 4A-B).

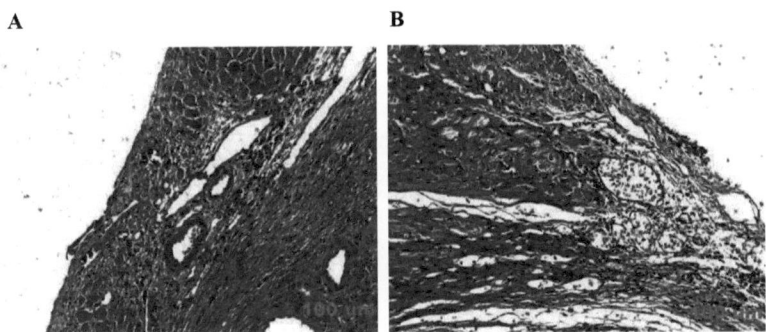

Figure 4 A-B. Representative images of H&E-stained paraffin sections of LV tissues from WT- and ERα-OE mice after MI. ERα-OE mice hearts showed an increased occurrence of vascular-like structures in the peri-infarct area. 20x magnification, scale bar 100μm.

In order to assess the nature of these vessel-like structures, we performed immunofluorescence double staining experiments using antibodies against *CD31* (*PECAM-1* or) for the staining of blood vessels, and against *LYVE-1* for the staining of lymphatic vessels. We observed that very few *CD31* and *LYVE-1* positive signals were expressed in the hearts of WT (Figure 4C, 4G) and ERα-OE sham mice (Figure 4E, 4I). After MI, predominately in the peri-infarct areas and to the lesser extent in the infarct areas, the signals for *CD31* and *LYVE-1* increased significantly in the peri-infarct and infarct areas in both female and male ERα-OE mice hearts, compared to their respective sham-operated mice (Figure 4E, 4F and Figure 4I, 4J). However, these effects were not observed in WT-mice hearts (Figure 4C, 4D and Figure 4G, 4H).

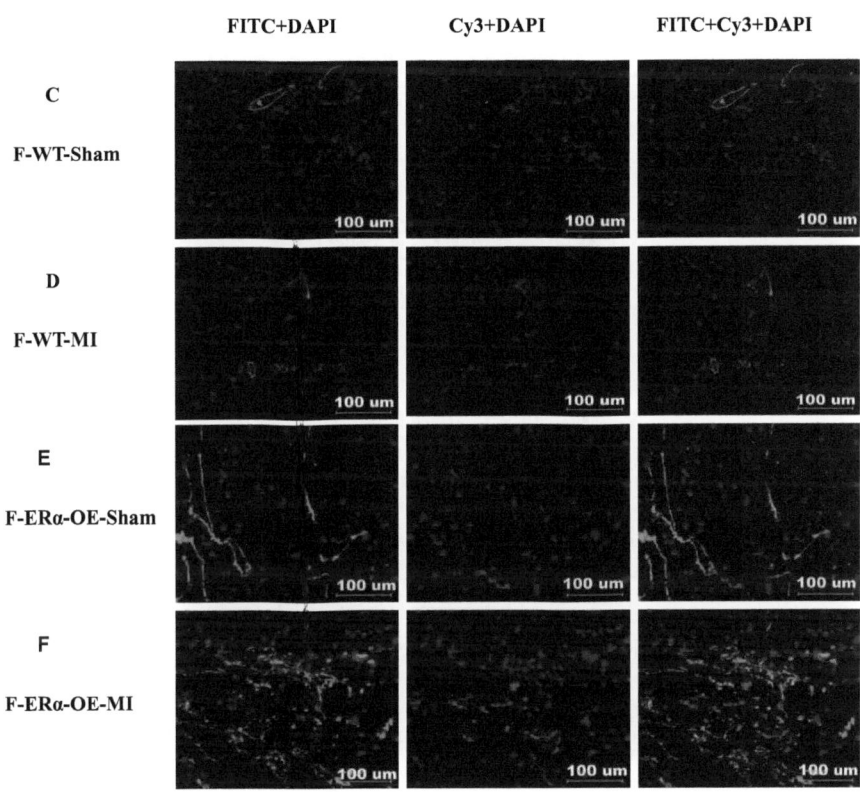

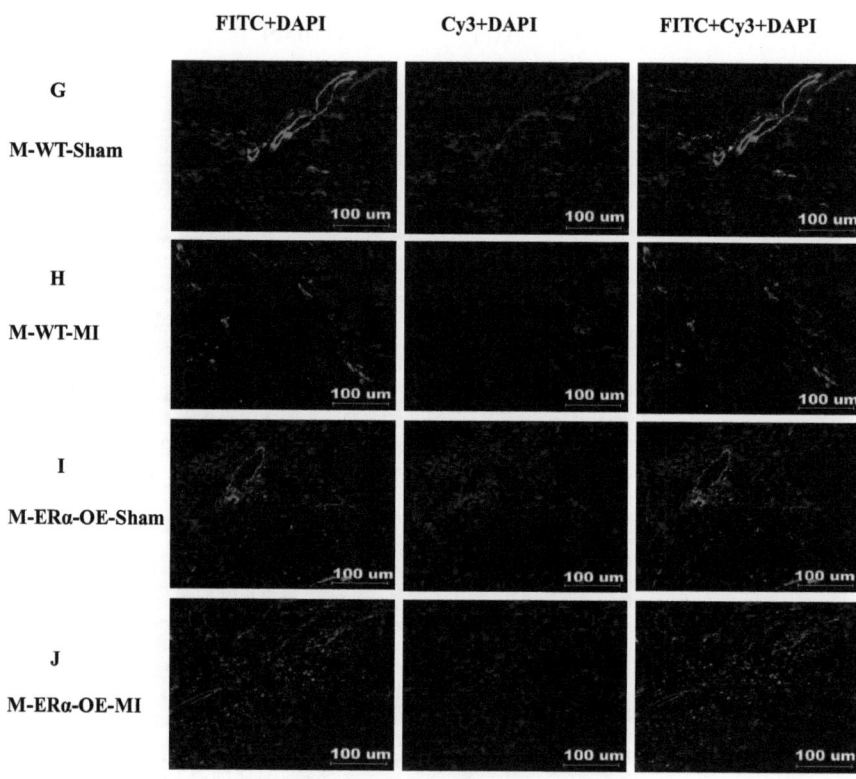

Figure 4 C-J. Representative immunofluorescence photographs of LV tissue in peri-infarct and infarct area from WT-female and male (C & D, G & H) and ERα-OE-female and male mice (E & F, I & J) 2 weeks after sham and MI operation using antibodies against *CD31* and *LYVE-1* (scale bar 100μm). *CD31*-positive vessels (FITC, green), *LYVE-1* positive vessels (Cy3, red), nuclei (DAPI, blue).

Additionally, we quantified areas of *LYVE-1-* and *CD31* expressing vessels in both sexes and genotype groups and among all treatment groups. As presented in Figures 5A and 5B, at the basal level, areas of *CD31-* and *LYVE-1* expressing vessels in both female and male ERα-OE mice hearts showed no significant changes compared to both female and male WT mice. After MI, in comparison to both female and male WT mice, female and male ERα-OE mice hearts showed significant increases in areas of *CD31-* and *LYVE-1* expressing vessels. Furthermore, areas of *CD31-* and *LYVE-1* expressing vessels significantly increased in both female and male ERα-OE mice after MI in comparison to their sham controls.

To confirm the increase of angiogenesis and lymphangiogenesis in ERα-OE mice hearts, we measured the expression of genes involved in these processes. In agreement with immunofluorescence analysis, the expression of *VEGF*, a key marker of angiogenesis, and *LYVE-1*, a key marker of lymphangiogenesis, were significantly increased in tissues from the infarct and peri-infarct area of female and male ERα-OE mice hearts compared with WT-mice (Figure 5C, 5D).

Taken together, ERα overexpression in cardiomyocytes accelerates both angiogenesis and lymphangiogenesis mainly in the border zones and to a lesser extent in the infarct areas in both sexes.

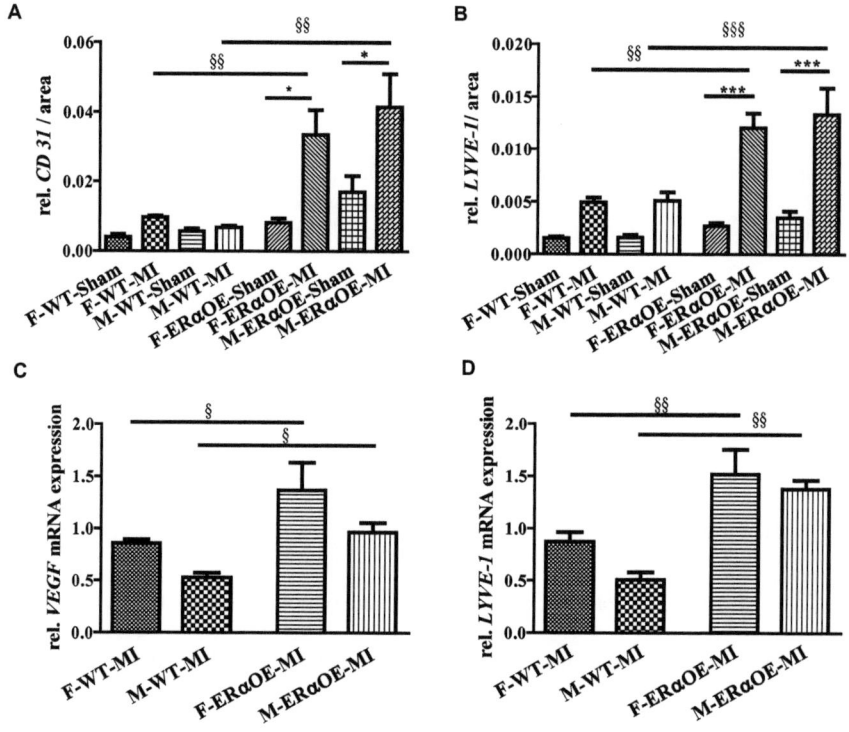

Figure 5A-B. Quantification of areas of *LYVE-1-* and *CD31* expressing vessels from Figure 4 C-J. Data expressed as mean±SEM of 3 to 4 animals per group. § for the genotype effect: females: $p<0.01$ (*LYVE-1*), $p<0.01$ (*CD31*); males: $p<0.001$ (*LYVE-1*), $p<0.01$ (*CD31*). * for MI effect: females: $p<0.001$ (*LYVE-1*), $p<0.05$ (*CD31*); males: $p<0.001$ (*LYVE-1*). **5C-D**, qRT-PCR analysis of the mRNA levels of *VEGF* and *LYVE-1* obtained from peri-infarct and infarct areas from WT- and ERα-OE mice. Data expressed as mean ±SEM of 5 to 6 animals per group. § for the genotype effect for each gene: females: $p<0.05$ (*VEGF*) and $p<0.01$ (*LYVE-1*); males: $p<0.05$ (*VEGF*) and 0.001 (*LYVE-1*).

4.3 ERα induces the phosphorylation of *JNK* signaling pathway only in female hearts after myocardial infarction

JNK1/3 is known as a positive regulator of the angiogenic process [91, 92]. Western blot analysis of LV extracts from both female and male WT- and ERα-OE mice showed that the phosphorylation level of *JNK* was significantly increased only in female ERα-OE mice hearts after MI (Figure 6).

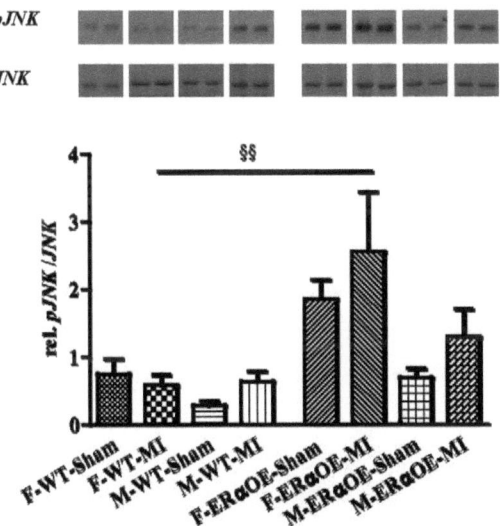

Figure 6. Expression of phosphorylated *JNK* (*pJNK*) was increased in only female ERα-OE mice hearts. Bar graph representing the quantitative western blot analysis of *pJNK* in LV tissues from female and male WT and ERα-OE mice. Data are expressed as a ratio of *pJNK* to *JNK*. Bars represent the mean ±SEM of 7 to 8 animals per group. §§ for genotype effect: $p<0.01$.

4.4 ERα attenuates collagen deposition after myocardial infarction only in female hearts

Proliferation of fibroblasts is essential for infarct healing and affects ventricular remodeling, one of the most important prognostic factors after myocardial infarction [93]. Fibrillar collagens play an important role in healing and remodeling after MI [94]. Therefore, we next assessed the effects of ERα overexpression on collagen deposition in the hearts of ERα-OE and WT-mice after MI using Sirius Red staining. As presented in Figure 7A, collagen staining of heart tissues from female and male WT- and ERα-OE mice showed a significant increase of collagen deposition in all groups after MI. However, hearts of female ERα-OE mice showed significantly less collagen deposition after MI, compared with female WT-mice (female ERα-OE vs. female WT, 0.13±0.01 vs. 0.26±0.02) (Figure 7B). Overall, ERα overexpression is associated with less fibrosis in female hearts, suggesting that the female ERα-OE hearts are less susceptible to MI-induced remodeling.

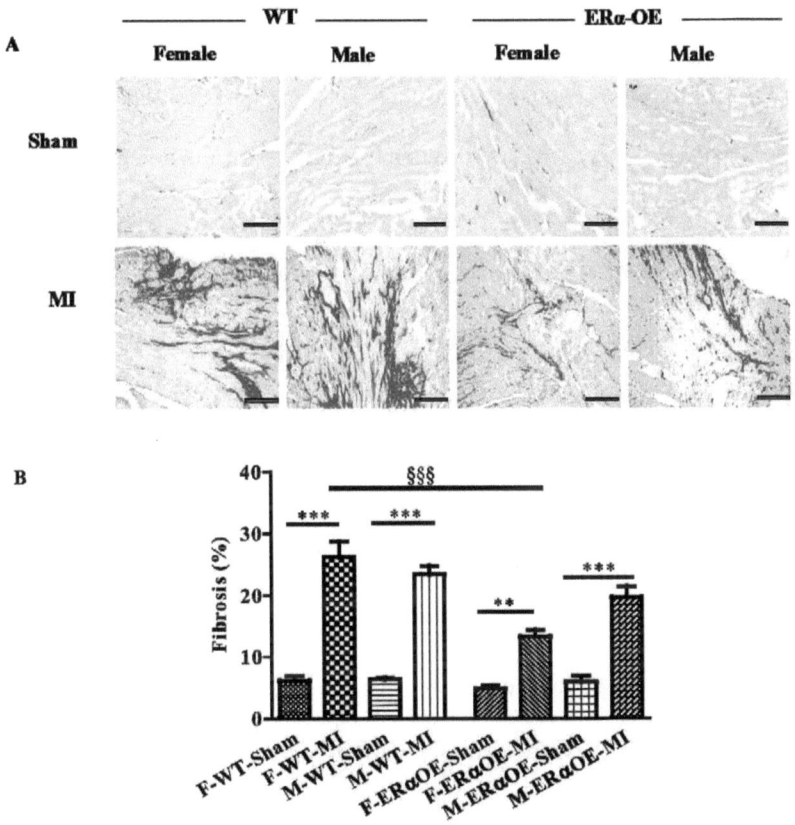

Figure 7A. Sirius Red staining of representative LV tissue (scale bar 100μm) and **7B.** Fibrosis quantification in WT- and ERα-OE mice 2 weeks after sham or MI. The level of interstitial collagen accumulation in female ERα-OE was significantly lower in comparison to female WT-mice after MI. Data expressed as mean ±SEM of 4 to 6 animals per group. § for the genotype effect: $p<0.001$. * for MI effect (MI vs. sham). WT-female: $p<0.001$ and ERα-OE-female $p<0.01$; WT-male: $p<0.001$ and ERα-OE -male $p<0.001$.

5 Discussion

In this study, we present novel insights into mechanisms that account for the ERα-dependent myocardial protection against myocardial injury, with more beneficial effects in female hearts. Using a transgenic mouse model with a cardiomyocyte-specific ERα-overexpression (ERα-OE), we first demonstrated that this was associated with an increase of LVM at the basal level in both female and male mice. After MI, the cardiomyocyte-specific ERα-OE inhibited changes in LV-volumes and wall thickness only in female mice. These beneficial effects in female ERα-OE hearts were associated with increased angiogenesis and lymphangiogenesis, attenuated ventricular fibrosis and enhanced *JNK* phosphorylation. Our study indicates that in the female sex, ERα in cardiomyocytes may have a therapeutic potential in the treatment of ischemic heart disease, leading to more efficient cardiac repair after ischemic injury.

5.1 Effects of ERα overexpression on the heart

To address the effect of ERα more precisely on cardiomyocyte following cardiac injury, we generated mice with a constitutive overexpression of ERα in cardiomyocytes. This unique model makes it possible to obtain new insights into ERα mediated cardioprotective mechanisms. The constitutive cardiomyocyte-specific ERα overexpression resulted in myocardial hypertrophy, associated with higher LVM and increased ventricular volumes. Consistent with

Discussion

these findings, in a parallel work in our group on this model (Dissertation of J. Leber, 2014), it has been shown that on microscopic examination of isolated cardiomyocytes, female and male ERα-OE displayed a significant increase in cardiomyocyte length, but not in cardiomyocyte width compared with WT-mice. Additionally, this study showed that there was no fibrosis, augmented expression of hypertrophy-associated genes natriuretic peptide precursor A (*Nppa*), natriuretic peptide precursor B (*Nppb*) and the ratio of myosin heavy chain 7 and 6 (*Myh7* /*Myh6*) in either sex at basal level (Dissertation of J. Leber, 2014). These are characteristics of an eccentric type of hypertrophy. Eccentric hypertrophy is predominantly characterized by the addition of sarcomeres in series, which leads to an increase in myocyte cell length and consequently increases the cardiac mass with increased chamber volume [95]. It has been observed in hearts during pregnancy or in athlete hearts after endurance training [95-98]. The eccentric hypertrophy induced by pregnancy or training is a physiological hypertrophy which is not typically associated with fibrosis [95-98].

The effects observed in our study may be due to direct effects of ERα as a transcription factor through the regulation of expression of hypertrophy-target genes, or indirectly due to hemodynamic alterations. My collaborator Joachim Leber also demonstrated a higher phosphorylation of ERα at *Ser118*, essential for transcriptional activation [99], as well as a greater translocation of ERα in the nuclei of ERα-OE mouse cardiomyocytes, indicating a functional role of ERα as a transcription factor in this model. Furthermore, in a previous study it was shown that the expression of hypertrophy-associated genes *Nppa*, *α-actinin* and *Cx43* is increased by E2-induced activation of ERα in a human cardiomyocyte-like cell line AC16 cells [100]. Therefore, the higher expression and activation of ERα could be an explanation for the increased expression of hypertrophy-associated genes in ERα-OE mice. It is also conceivable that the higher expression of *Nppa*, *Nppb* and *Myh7* in the LV of ERα-OE is a response to increased cardiomyocyte stretch due to increased cardiomyocyte length, as reported elsewhere [101-104].

5.2 Effects of ERα overexpression following myocardial infarction

5.2.1 ERα overexpression enhances neovascularization after myocardial infarction

Following MI, hearts of female ERα-OE mice did not exhibit accelerated post-infarct remodeling. Compared to WT and male ERα-OE mice, in female ERα-OE hearts systolic and diastolic volumes were not increased and LV wall thickness not significantly decreased after MI. These phenomena may lead to reduced wall stress in female ERα-OE hearts after MI, thus attenuating the adverse consequences of remodeling. In this study, we also provide evidence that cardiomyocyte-specific ERα overexpression promotes angiogenesis and lymphangiogenesis in the heart after MI in both sexes.

Angiogenesis and lymphangiogenesis are associated with post-infarct remodeling and have important implications for prognosis following MI [105, 106]. Angiogenesis and lymphangiogenesis represent the formation of new blood vessels and new lymphatic vessels by cellular outgrowth from existing microvessels [107, 108] and occur as part of the natural healing process following ischemic injury. In this respect, the mRNA expression of angiogenesis and lymphangiogenesis markers *VEGF* and *LYVE-1* and the area of both *CD31-* and *LYVE-1* expressing vessels were significantly increased in the infarct and peri-infarct tissues of ERα-OE mice. This indicates that ERα induces angiogenesis and lymphangiogenesis in the heart after MI. The effects of E2 in different tissues on angiogenesis, mainly mediated by ERα, have been demonstrated by findings in the ERKO mice [109-112], in which angiogenesis is impaired. Furthermore, it has been shown that ERα antagonists can inhibit angiogenesis [113], while ERα-agonist can promote angiogenesis [114]. These data reveal that ERα plays an important role in the regulation of angiogenesis.

In experimental studies, Banai et al. [115] suggested that VEGF leads to myocardial neovascularization in the process of MI. Ferrarini et al. [116] showed that VEGF was diffusely expressed in the surviving cardiomyocytes and enhanced both angiogenesis and cardiomyocyte viability in infarcted myocardium. Ishikawa et al. [106] suggested that, besides other contributors, VEGF is critical for lymphangiogenesis in the healing area of MI. Previous studies have demonstrated that VEGF can be regulated by E2 in different organs, including the myocardium [117-120]. Jesmin et al. [77] clearly demonstrated that the absence or deficiency of functional ER disrupts levels of VEGF and components of its signaling machinery (VEGF receptors, eNOS, and Akt) in female mouse hearts. Such disruptive effects, in addition to reduced total coronary capillary density, were more profound in ERKO compared with WT mice [120]. Hamada et al. [121] also suggested that VEGF was significantly downregulated in ERKO mice compared with WT mice after cardiac ischemic injury. These studies speculated that this estrogenic effect is most probably mediated through activation of ERα, since the absence or deficiency of functional ERα leads to the reduction of expression level of VEGF and reduced coronary capillary density in female mouse hearts [77]. Additionally, it has been reported that E2-activated ER inhibits the expression and secretion of Thrombospondin-1, a negative regulator of angiogenesis, in human umbilical vein endothelial cells through activation of JNK in a non-genomic manner [122]. In line with this data we observed an increased phosphorylation of *JNK* (*pJNK*) only in the hearts of female ERα-OE mice after MI. Therefore, we suppose that a higher baseline of endogenous E2 in females, compared to males, led to preferential activation of *JNK* in female ERα-OE cardiomyocytes. The E2/ERα mediated *JNK*-activation in this study could be either mediated by increased expression of cardiomyocytes-derived VEGF in a paracrine manner, as shown in vascular endothelial cells [91, 92], or it demonstrates an additional mechanism independent of VEGF in the female ERα-OE mouse heart.

Experimental evidence suggests that E2 also plays important roles in lymphangiogenesis. Brown et al. [123] have demonstrated that E2 is likely to regulate ovarian lymphangiogenesis via ERα on the lymphatic endothelium. However, so far it is not clear to what extent ERα affects lymphangiogenesis in the heart after MI. To the best of our knowledge, this study is the first work that shows the involvement of ERα in the enhancement of lymphangiogenesis after MI. Like angiogenesis, lymphangiogenesis also plays an important role in cardiac repair after MI. The principal physiological function of the lymphatic vasculature is to take up fluid leaking out of blood capillaries into interstitial spaces in the tissue, and to return it to the blood circulation [124, 125]. Failures in this system result in lymphedema [108, 126, 127]. A previous study [128] described that impairment of cardiac lymphatic flow due to MI results in excess fluid accumulation and formation of cardiac lymphedema. Ullal et al. [129] also found that blocking cardiac lymph flow led to valvular lymphatic vessel dilation, myxoid deposition, and mild fibrosis. Although the underlying mechanism of cardiac dysfunction caused by cardiac lymph flow impairment has not been fully explored, there are some promising studies about the beneficial effect on heart function by active promotion of lymph fluid drainage in the impaired heart. Szlavy et al. [130] studied cardiac lymph flow after MI in a dog model, and found that cardiac lymph flow decreased shortly after MI and cardiac lymphatic filling was decreased in the ischemic zone. Hyaluronidase acted as lymphagogue, maintained lymphatic vascular patency and was found to prevent lymphatic occlusion as well as collapse in this model. Some similar studies also described hyaluronidase as preventing cardiac injury from myocardial ischemia [131, 132] or I/R [133] in dog models.

Based on our data and data from literature, it is conceivable that ERα-OE may, at least partly, prevent myocardial edema and cardiac dysfunction via improving cardiac lymph flow after MI in female mice [132].

5.2.2 ERα overexpression affects cardiac remodeling following myocardial infarction

The fact that progressive myocardial fibrosis is a pathological feature associated with cardiac remodeling following MI has been well documented. Cardiac remodeling following MI involves complex biochemical, molecular and morphological alterations in both ischemic and remote myocardial area. This remodeling involves phenotypic changes in the myocytes as well as in the extracellular matrix, which results in myocardial fibrosis as a consequence of an imbalance between its production and degradation [134]. Progressive cardiac fibrosis contributes to an increase in cardiac muscle stiffness, leading to cardiac dysfunction [135]. Hypoxia has been proposed to be pro-fibrotic in the heart via induction of hypoxia-inducible factor (HIF)-1α, which may explain the increased fibrosis in cardiac allograft remodeling [136]. Additionally, Laine et al. [137] found that myocardial fibrosis is also associated with cardiac edema after cardiac injury, such as MI. Casley-Smith et al. [138] believed that the presence of high-protein concentration within edema stimulates the deposition of fibrotic material. Therefore, anti-hypoxia and reduced cardiac edema are potential therapeutic targets in fibrosis and wound healing. Indeed, lymphangiogenesis in the peri-infarct area improves cardiac lymph flow leading to reduced cardiac edema, thereby reducing a trigger for the development of interstitial fibrosis [93]. Davis et al. [139] demonstrated in a rat model that chronic myocardial edema was accompanied by increased mRNA levels of collagen types I and III, resulting in increased LV collagen deposition. In our study, although both female and male ERα-OE mice displayed increased angiogenesis and lymphangiogenesis, only female ERα-OE mice exhibited significantly reduced collagen expression after MI. These data are further supported by a recent study [140] showing that ERα is significantly involved in the inhibition of cardiac fibrosis in female mice. The increased angiogenesis/lymphangiogenesis and attenuated fibrosis in female ERα-OE following MI could be one explanation for the phenomenon that hearts of female ERα-OE mice did not exhibit accelerated or adverse post-infarct remodeling, indicated by maintained systolic and diastolic volumes and LV wall thickness after MI. However, in male ERα-OE mice despite the higher angiogenesis/lymphangiogenesis, the activation of JNK-pathway and attenuation of fibrosis were not as pronounced as in female ERα-OE mice after MI. It seems that in male ERα-OE mice the activation angiogenesis/lymphangiogenesis alone is not sufficient to contribute to the improved cardiac remodeling.

Overall, this is the first report showing that cardiomyocyte-specific overexpression of ERα (ERα-OE) leads to spontaneous development of cardiac hypertrophy in mice. After MI, ERα-OE leads to higher neovascularization in the peri-infarct and infarct area. Only female ERα-OE mice exhibited improved post-infarct remodeling. Compared to WT and male ERα-OE mice, in female ERα-OE hearts, systolic and diastolic volume was not increased and LV wall thickness was not significantly decreased after MI. These phenomena suggest that cardiomyocyte-specific ERα provides cardioprotection in female mice by enhancing vascular structure and function, and attenuation of cardiac remodeling in a paracrine fashion in response to cardiac ischemic injury (Figure 8).

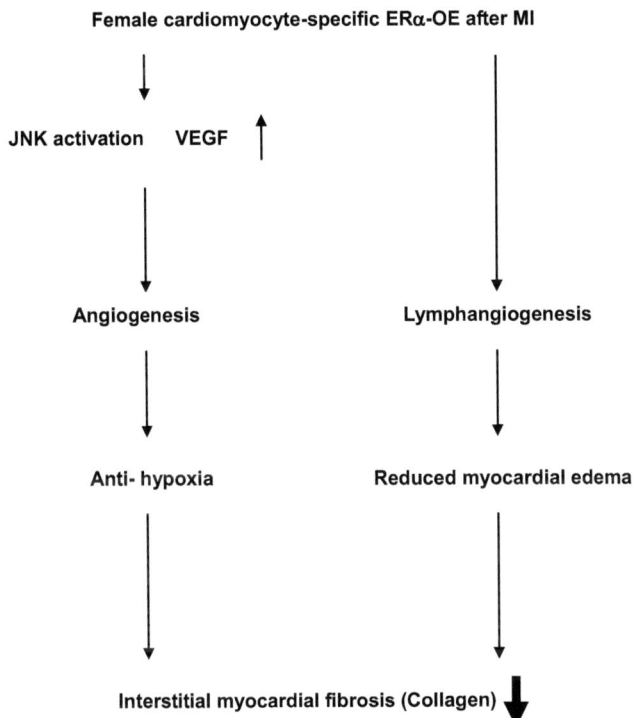

Figure 8. Cardiomyocyte-specific ERα provides cardioprotection in ERα-OE female mice by enhancing angiogenesis and lymphangiogenesis, and attenuation of cardiac fibrosis, leading to less accelerated cardiac remodeling after MI.

6 Bibliography

1. World Health Organisation,"cardiovascular diseases (CVDs). 2013; Available from: (Accessed March 12 , 2013, at http://www.who.int/mediacentre/factsheets/fs317/en/).

2. Myers, L. and S. Mendis, Cardiovascular disease research output in WHO priority areas between 2002 and 2011. J Epidemiol Glob Health, 2014. 4(1): p. 23-8.

3. Bhatia, S.K., Biomaterials for clinical applications. 2010, New York: Springer. p. 23. ISBN 9781441969200.

4. Thygesen, K., et al., Universal definition of myocardial infarction. J Am Coll Cardiol, 2007. 50(22): p. 2173-95.

5. Jugdutt, B.I., Ischemia/Infarction. Heart Fail Clin, 2012. 8(1): p. 43-51.

6. Herskowitz A1, C.S., Ansari AA, Wesselingh S., Cytokine mRNA expression in postischemic/reperfused myocardium. Am J Pathol, 1995 Feb. 146(2): p. 419-28.

7. Ferdinandy, P., R. Schulz, and G.F. Baxter, Interaction of cardiovascular risk factors with myocardial ischemia/reperfusion injury, preconditioning, and postconditioning. Pharmacol Rev, 2007. 59(4): p. 418-58.

8. Frank, A., et al., Myocardial ischemia reperfusion injury: from basic science to clinical bedside. Semin Cardiothorac Vasc Anesth, 2012. 16(3): p. 123-32.

9. Vanlangenakker N1, V.B.T., Krysko DV, Festjens N, Vandenabeele P., Molecular mechanisms and pathophysiology of necrotic cell death. Curr Mol Med, 2008 May. 8(3): p. 207-20.

10. Buja, L.M., Myocardial ischemia and reperfusion injury. Cardiovasc Pathol, 2005. 14(4): p. 170-5.

11. Abbate, A., et al., Increased myocardial apoptosis in patients with unfavorable left ventricular remodeling and early symptomatic post-infarction heart failure. J Am Coll Cardiol, 2003. 41(5): p. 753-60.

12. Fan, D., et al., Cardiac fibroblasts, fibrosis and extracellular matrix remodeling in heart disease. Fibrogenesis Tissue Repair, 2012. 5(1): p. 15.

13. Stefanon, I., et al., Left and right ventricle late remodeling following myocardial infarction in rats. PLoS One, 2013. 8(5): p. e64986.

14. Rouillard, A.D. and J.W. Holmes, Mechanical regulation of fibroblast migration and collagen remodelling in healing myocardial infarcts. J Physiol, 2012. 590(Pt 18): p. 4585-602.

15. Zentilin, L., et al., Cardiomyocyte VEGFR-1 activation by VEGF-B induces

compensatory hypertrophy and preserves cardiac function after myocardial infarction. FASEB J, 2010. 24(5): p. 1467-78.

16. Kumamoto, H., et al., Beneficial effect of myocardial angiogenesis on cardiac remodeling process by amlodipine and MCI-154. Am J Physiol, 1999. 276(4 Pt 2): p. H1117-23.

17. Vandoorne, K., et al., Chronic Akt1 deficiency attenuates adverse remodeling and enhances angiogenesis after myocardial infarction. Circ Cardiovasc Imaging, 2013. 6(6): p. 992-1000.

18. Reckelhoff, J.F. and C. Maric, Sex and gender differences in cardiovascular-renal physiology and pathophysiology. Steroids, 2010. 75(11): p. 745-6.

19. Kim, E.S. and V. Menon, Status of women in cardiovascular clinical trials. Arterioscler Thromb Vasc Biol, 2009. 29(3): p. 279-83.

20. Coylewright, M., J.F. Reckelhoff, and P. Ouyang, Menopause and hypertension: an age-old debate. Hypertension, 2008. 51(4): p. 952-9.

21. Bittner, V., Menopause, age, and cardiovascular risk: a complex relationship. J Am Coll Cardiol, 2009. 54(25): p. 2374-5.

22. Crabbe, D.L., et al., Gender differences in post-infarction hypertrophy in

end-stage failing hearts. J Am Coll Cardiol, 2003. 41(2): p. 300-6.

23. Hayward, C.S., R.P. Kelly, and P. Collins, The roles of gender, the menopause and hormone replacement on cardiovascular function. Cardiovasc Res, 2000. 46(1): p. 28-49.

24. Carroll, J.D., et al., Sex-associated differences in left ventricular function in aortic stenosis of the elderly. Circulation, 1992. 86(4): p. 1099-107.

25. Regitz-Zagrosek, V., Therapeutic implications of the gender-specific aspects of cardiovascular disease. Nat Rev Drug Discov, 2006. 5(5): p. 425-38.

26. Korhonen, J. and P. Koskinen, Acute myocardial infarction. A study of the sex distribution, immediate mortality, age distribution, incidence of hypertension and diabetes, and the effect of the seasons in a series of 376 cases. Ann Med Intern Fenn, 1960. 49: p. 247-54.

27. Kannel, W.B., et al., Menopause and risk of cardiovascular disease: the Framingham study. Ann Intern Med, 1976. 85(4): p. 447-52.

28. Grodstein, F. and M. Stampfer, The epidemiology of coronary heart disease and estrogen replacement in postmenopausal women. Prog Cardiovasc Dis, 1995. 38(3): p. 199-210.

29. Hulley, S., et al., Randomized trial of estrogen plus progestin for secondary

prevention of coronary heart disease in postmenopausal women. Heart and Estrogen/progestin Replacement Study (HERS) Research Group. JAMA, 1998. 280(7): p. 605-13.

30. Hulley, S. and D. Grady, Postmenopausal hormone treatment. JAMA, 2009. 301(23): p. 2493-5.

31. Luczak, E.D. and L.A. Leinwand, Sex-based cardiac physiology. Annu Rev Physiol, 2009. 71: p. 1-18.

32. Anisimov, V.N., et al., Gender differences in metformin effect on aging, life span and spontaneous tumorigenesis in 129/Sv mice. Aging (Albany NY), 2010. 2(12): p. 945-58.

33. Dedkov, E.I., et al., Coronary vessels and cardiac myocytes of middle-aged rats demonstrate regional sex-specific adaptation in response to postmyocardial infarction remodeling. Biol Sex Differ, 2014. 5(1): p. 1.

34. van Eickels, M., et al., 17beta-estradiol attenuates the development of pressure-overload hypertrophy. Circulation, 2001. 104(12): p. 1419-23.

35. Hale, S.L., Y. Birnbaum, and R.A. Kloner, beta-Estradiol, but not alpha-estradiol, reduced myocardial necrosis in rabbits after ischemia and reperfusion. Am Heart J, 1996. 132(2 Pt 1): p. 258-62.

36. Kim, J.K. and E.R. Levin, Estrogen signaling in the cardiovascular system. Nucl Recept Signal, 2006. 4: p. e013.

37. Thompson, L.P., G. Pinkas, and C.P. Weiner, Chronic 17beta-estradiol replacement increases nitric oxide-mediated vasodilation of guinea pig coronary microcirculation. Circulation, 2000. 102(4): p. 445-51.

38. Guo, X., et al., Estrogen induces vascular wall dilation: mediation through kinase signaling to nitric oxide and estrogen receptors alpha and beta. J Biol Chem, 2005. 280(20): p. 19704-10.

39. Beer, S., et al., Susceptibility to cardiac ischemia/reperfusion injury is modulated by chronic estrogen status. J Cardiovasc Pharmacol, 2002. 40(3): p. 420-8.

40. Xu, Y., et al., Cardioprotection by chronic estrogen or superoxide dismutase mimetic treatment in the aged female rat. Am J Physiol Heart Circ Physiol, 2004. 287(1): p. H165-71.

41. Shlipak, M.G., et al., Hormone therapy and in-hospital survival after myocardial infarction in postmenopausal women. Circulation, 2001. 104(19): p. 2300-4.

42. Kim, J.K., et al., Estrogen prevents cardiomyocyte apoptosis through inhibition of reactive oxygen species and differential regulation of p38

kinase isoforms. J Biol Chem, 2006. 281(10): p. 6760-7.

43. Kolodgie, F.D., et al., Myocardial protection of contractile function after global ischemia by physiologic estrogen replacement in the ovariectomized rat. J Mol Cell Cardiol, 1997. 29(9): p. 2403-14.

44. Jeanes, H.L., et al., Oestrogen-mediated cardioprotection following ischaemia and reperfusion is mimicked by an oestrogen receptor (ER)alpha agonist and unaffected by an ER beta antagonist. J Endocrinol, 2008. 197(3): p. 493-501.

45. Squadrito, F., et al., 17Beta-oestradiol reduces cardiac leukocyte accumulation in myocardial ischaemia reperfusion injury in rat. Eur J Pharmacol, 1997. 335(2-3): p. 185-92.

46. Scheuer, J., et al., Effects of gonadectomy and hormonal replacement on rat hearts. Circ Res, 1987. 61(1): p. 12-9.

47. Babiker, F.A., et al., 17beta-estradiol antagonizes cardiomyocyte hypertrophy by autocrine/paracrine stimulation of a guanylyl cyclase A receptor-cyclic guanosine monophosphate-dependent protein kinase pathway. Circulation, 2004. 109(2): p. 269-76.

48. Cui, Y.H., et al., 17 beta-estradiol attenuates pressure overload-induced myocardial hypertrophy through regulating caveolin-3 protein in

ovariectomized female rats. Mol Biol Rep, 2011. 38(8): p. 4885-92.

49. Patten, R.D., et al., 17 Beta-estradiol differentially affects left ventricular and cardiomyocyte hypertrophy following myocardial infarction and pressure overload. J Card Fail, 2008. 14(3): p. 245-53.

50. Krasinski, K., et al., Estradiol accelerates functional endothelial recovery after arterial injury. Circulation, 1997. 95(7): p. 1768-72.

51. Mendelsohn, M.E. and R.H. Karas, Molecular and cellular basis of cardiovascular gender differences. Science, 2005. 308(5728): p. 1583-7.

52. Toft, D. and J. Gorski, A receptor molecule for estrogens: isolation from the rat uterus and preliminary characterization. Proc Natl Acad Sci U S A, 1966. 55(6): p. 1574-81.

53. Jensen, E.V., et al., A two-step mechanism for the interaction of estradiol with rat uterus. Proc Natl Acad Sci U S A, 1968. 59(2): p. 632-8.

54. Kuiper, G.G., et al., Cloning of a novel receptor expressed in rat prostate and ovary. Proc Natl Acad Sci U S A, 1996. 93(12): p. 5925-30.

55. Mosselman, S., J. Polman, and R. Dijkema, ER beta: identification and characterization of a novel human estrogen receptor. FEBS Lett, 1996. 392(1): p. 49-53.

56. Nilsson, S. and J.A. Gustafsson, Estrogen receptor action. Crit Rev Eukaryot Gene Expr, 2002. 12(4): p. 237-57.

57. Karas, R.H., B.L. Patterson, and M.E. Mendelsohn, Human vascular smooth muscle cells contain functional estrogen receptor. Circulation, 1994. 89(5): p. 1943-50.

58. Kim-Schulze, S., et al., Expression of an estrogen receptor by human coronary artery and umbilical vein endothelial cells. Circulation, 1996. 94(6): p. 1402-7.

59. Grohe, C., et al., Cardiac myocytes and fibroblasts contain functional estrogen receptors. FEBS Lett, 1997. 416(1): p. 107-12.

60. Nordmeyer, J., et al., Upregulation of myocardial estrogen receptors in human aortic stenosis. Circulation, 2004. 110(20): p. 3270-5.

61. Groten, T., et al., 17 beta-estradiol transiently disrupts adherens junctions in endothelial cells. FASEB J, 2005. 19(10): p. 1368-70.

62. Mahmoodzadeh, S., et al., Estrogen receptor alpha up-regulation and redistribution in human heart failure. FASEB J, 2006. 20(7): p. 926-34.

63. Ropero, A.B., et al., Heart estrogen receptor alpha: distinct membrane and nuclear distribution patterns and regulation by estrogen. J Mol Cell Cardiol,

2006. 41(3): p. 496-510.

64. Aranda, A. and A. Pascual, Nuclear hormone receptors and gene expression. Physiol Rev, 2001. 81(3): p. 1269-304.

65. Marino, M., P. Galluzzo, and P. Ascenzi, Estrogen signaling multiple pathways to impact gene transcription. Curr Genomics, 2006. 7(8): p. 497-508.

66. Arias-Loza, P.A., V. Jazbutyte, and T. Pelzer, Genetic and pharmacologic strategies to determine the function of estrogen receptor alpha and estrogen receptor beta in cardiovascular system. Gend Med, 2008. 5 Suppl A: p. S34-45.

67. Deschamps, A.M., E. Murphy, and J. Sun, Estrogen receptor activation and cardioprotection in ischemia reperfusion injury. Trends Cardiovasc Med, 2010. 20(3): p. 73-8.

68. Zhai, P., et al., Myocardial ischemia-reperfusion injury in estrogen receptor-alpha knockout and wild-type mice. Am J Physiol Heart Circ Physiol, 2000. 278(5): p. H1640-7.

69. Wang, M., et al., Estrogen receptor-alpha mediates acute myocardial protection in females. Am J Physiol Heart Circ Physiol, 2006. 290(6): p. H2204-9.

70. Babiker, F.A., et al., Oestrogen modulates cardiac ischaemic remodelling through oestrogen receptor-specific mechanisms. Acta Physiol (Oxf), 2007. 189(1): p. 23-31.

71. Booth, E.A., N.R. Obeid, and B.R. Lucchesi, Activation of estrogen receptor-alpha protects the in vivo rabbit heart from ischemia-reperfusion injury. Am J Physiol Heart Circ Physiol, 2005. 289(5): p. H2039-47.

72. Nikolic, I., et al., Treatment with an estrogen receptor-beta-selective agonist is cardioprotective. J Mol Cell Cardiol, 2007. 42(4): p. 769-80.

73. Losordo, D.W., et al., Variable expression of the estrogen receptor in normal and atherosclerotic coronary arteries of premenopausal women. Circulation, 1994. 89(4): p. 1501-10.

74. Post, W.S., et al., Methylation of the estrogen receptor gene is associated with aging and atherosclerosis in the cardiovascular system. Cardiovasc Res, 1999. 43(4): p. 985-91.

75. Novotny, J.L., et al., Rapid estrogen receptor-alpha activation improves ischemic tolerance in aged female rats through a novel protein kinase C epsilon-dependent mechanism. Endocrinology, 2009. 150(2): p. 889-96.

76. Vornehm, N.D., et al., Acute postischemic treatment with estrogen receptor-alpha agonist or estrogen receptor-beta agonist improves

myocardial recovery. Surgery, 2009. 146(2): p. 145-54.

77. Jesmin, S., et al., VEGF signaling is disrupted in the hearts of mice lacking estrogen receptor alpha. Eur J Pharmacol, 2010. 641(2-3): p. 168-78.

78. Takemura, G. and H. Fujiwara, Role of apoptosis in remodeling after myocardial infarction. Pharmacol Ther, 2004. 104(1): p. 1-16.

79. Hruska, K.S., et al., Conditional over-expression of estrogen receptor alpha in a transgenic mouse model. Transgenic Res, 2002. 11(4): p. 361-72.

80. Yu, Z., C.S. Redfern, and G.I. Fishman, Conditional transgene expression in the heart. Circ Res, 1996. 79(4): p. 691-7.

81. Borst, O., et al., Methods employed for induction and analysis of experimental myocardial infarction in mice. Cell Physiol Biochem, 2011. 28(1): p. 1-12.

82. Ytrehus, K., The ischemic heart--experimental models. Pharmacol Res, 2000. 42(3): p. 193-203.

83. Liu, Y.H., et al., Chronic heart failure induced by coronary artery ligation in Lewis inbred rats. Am J Physiol, 1997. 272(2 Pt 2): p. H722-7.

84. Yang, X.P., et al., Echocardiographic assessment of cardiac function in conscious and anesthetized mice. Am J Physiol, 1999. 277(5 Pt 2): p.

H1967-74.

85. Coatney, R.W., Ultrasound imaging: principles and applications in rodent research. ILAR J, 2001. 42(3): p. 233-47.

86. Collins, K.A., et al., Accuracy of echocardiographic estimates of left ventricular mass in mice. Am J Physiol Heart Circ Physiol, 2001. 280(5): p. H1954-62.

87. Benavides-Vallve, C., et al., New strategies for echocardiographic evaluation of left ventricular function in a mouse model of long-term myocardial infarction. PLoS One, 2012. 7(7): p. e41691.

88. Zhou, Z., et al., Antibody against murine PECAM-1 inhibits tumor angiogenesis in mice. Angiogenesis, 1999. 3(2): p. 181-8.

89. Karunamuni, G., et al., Expression of lymphatic markers during avian and mouse cardiogenesis. Anat Rec (Hoboken), 2010. 293(2): p. 259-70.

90. Schmittgen, T.D. and K.J. Livak, Analyzing real-time PCR data by the comparative C(T) method. Nat Protoc, 2008. 3(6): p. 1101-8.

91. Uchida, C., et al., JNK as a positive regulator of angiogenic potential in endothelial cells. Cell Biol Int, 2008. 32(7): p. 769-76.

92. Wu, G., et al., Involvement of COX-2 in VEGF-induced angiogenesis via

P38 and JNK pathways in vascular endothelial cells. Cardiovasc Res, 2006. 69(2): p. 512-9.

93. Weber, K.T., et al., Remodeling and reparation of the cardiovascular system. J Am Coll Cardiol, 1992. 20(1): p. 3-16.

94. Pfeffer, M.A. and E. Braunwald, Ventricular remodeling after myocardial infarction. Experimental observations and clinical implications. Circulation, 1990. 81(4): p. 1161-72.

95. Dorn, G.W., 2nd, The fuzzy logic of physiological cardiac hypertrophy. Hypertension, 2007. 49(5): p. 962-70.

96. Eghbali, M., et al., Molecular and functional signature of heart hypertrophy during pregnancy. Circ Res, 2005. 96(11): p. 1208-16.

97. Fernandes, T., U.P. Soci, and E.M. Oliveira, Eccentric and concentric cardiac hypertrophy induced by exercise training: microRNAs and molecular determinants. Braz J Med Biol Res, 2011. 44(9): p. 836-47.

98. Zhang, Y., K. Novak, and S. Kaufman, Atrial natriuretic factor release during pregnancy in rats. J Physiol, 1995. 488 (Pt 2): p. 509-14.

99. Lannigan, D.A., Estrogen receptor phosphorylation. Steroids, 2003. 68(1): p. 1-9.

100. Mahmoodzadeh, S., et al., 17beta-Estradiol-induced interaction of ERalpha with NPPA regulates gene expression in cardiomyocytes. Cardiovasc Res, 2012. 96(3): p. 411-21.

101. Ellmers, L.J., et al., Ventricular expression of natriuretic peptides in Npr1(-/-) mice with cardiac hypertrophy and fibrosis. Am J Physiol Heart Circ Physiol, 2002. 283(2): p. H707-14.

102. Holtwick, R., et al., Pressure-independent cardiac hypertrophy in mice with cardiomyocyte-restricted inactivation of the atrial natriuretic peptide receptor guanylyl cyclase-A. J Clin Invest, 2003. 111(9): p. 1399-407.

103. Molkentin, J.D. and G.W. Dorn, 2nd, Cytoplasmic signaling pathways that regulate cardiac hypertrophy. Annu Rev Physiol, 2001. 63: p. 391-426.

104. Wagner, N., et al., Peroxisome proliferator-activated receptor beta stimulation induces rapid cardiac growth and angiogenesis via direct activation of calcineurin. Cardiovasc Res, 2009. 83(1): p. 61-71.

105. Fraccarollo, D., P. Galuppo, and J. Bauersachs, Novel therapeutic approaches to post-infarction remodelling. Cardiovasc Res, 2012. 94(2): p. 293-303.

106. Ishikawa, Y., et al., Lymphangiogenesis in myocardial remodelling after infarction. Histopathology, 2007. 51(3): p. 345-53.

107. Battegay, E.J., Angiogenesis: mechanistic insights, neovascular diseases, and therapeutic prospects. J Mol Med (Berl), 1995. 73(7): p. 333-46.

108. Norrmen, C., et al., Biological basis of therapeutic lymphangiogenesis. Circulation, 2011. 123(12): p. 1335-51.

109. Ardelt, A.A., et al., Estradiol regulates angiopoietin-1 mRNA expression through estrogen receptor-alpha in a rodent experimental stroke model. Stroke, 2005. 36(2): p. 337-41.

110. Brouchet, L., et al., Estradiol accelerates reendothelialization in mouse carotid artery through estrogen receptor-alpha but not estrogen receptor-beta. Circulation, 2001. 103(3): p. 423-8.

111. Johns, A., et al., Disruption of estrogen receptor gene prevents 17 beta estradiol-induced angiogenesis in transgenic mice. Endocrinology, 1996. 137(10): p. 4511-3.

112. Pare, G., et al., Estrogen receptor-alpha mediates the protective effects of estrogen against vascular injury. Circ Res, 2002. 90(10): p. 1087-92.

113. Gagliardi, A. and D.C. Collins, Inhibition of angiogenesis by antiestrogens. Cancer Res, 1993. 53(3): p. 533-5.

114. Zaitseva, M., et al., Estrogen receptor-alpha agonists promote angiogenesis

in human myometrial microvascular endothelial cells. J Soc Gynecol Investig, 2004. 11(8): p. 529-35.

115. Banai, S., et al., Upregulation of vascular endothelial growth factor expression induced by myocardial ischaemia: implications for coronary angiogenesis. Cardiovasc Res, 1994. 28(8): p. 1176-9.

116. Ferrarini, M., et al., Adeno-associated virus-mediated transduction of VEGF165 improves cardiac tissue viability and functional recovery after permanent coronary occlusion in conscious dogs. Circ Res, 2006. 98(7): p. 954-61.

117. Buteau-Lozano, H., et al., Transcriptional regulation of vascular endothelial growth factor by estradiol and tamoxifen in breast cancer cells: a complex interplay between estrogen receptors alpha and beta. Cancer Res, 2002. 62(17): p. 4977-84.

118. Gargett, C.E., et al., 17Beta-estradiol up-regulates vascular endothelial growth factor receptor-2 expression in human myometrial microvascular endothelial cells: role of estrogen receptor-alpha and -beta. J Clin Endocrinol Metab, 2002. 87(9): p. 4341-9.

119. Morales, D.E., et al., Estrogen promotes angiogenic activity in human umbilical vein endothelial cells in vitro and in a murine model. Circulation,

1995. 91(3): p. 755-63.

120. Jesmin, S., et al., In vivo estrogen manipulations on coronary capillary network and angiogenic molecule expression in middle-aged female rats. Arterioscler Thromb Vasc Biol, 2002. 22(10): p. 1591-7.

121. Hamada, H., et al., Estrogen receptors alpha and beta mediate contribution of bone marrow-derived endothelial progenitor cells to functional recovery after myocardial infarction. Circulation, 2006. 114(21): p. 2261-70.

122. Sengupta, K., et al., Thombospondin-1 disrupts estrogen-induced endothelial cell proliferation and migration and its expression is suppressed by estradiol. Mol Cancer Res, 2004. 2(3): p. 150-8.

123. Brown, H.M., R.L. Robker, and D.L. Russell, Development and hormonal regulation of the ovarian lymphatic vasculature. Endocrinology, 2010. 151(11): p. 5446-55.

124. Cueni, L.N. and M. Detmar, The lymphatic system in health and disease. Lymphat Res Biol, 2008. 6(3-4): p. 109-22.

125. Wang, Y. and G. Oliver, Current views on the function of the lymphatic vasculature in health and disease. Genes Dev, 2010. 24(19): p. 2115-26.

126. Kim, H. and D.J. Dumont, Molecular mechanisms in lymphangiogenesis:

model systems and implications in human disease. Clin Genet, 2003. 64(4): p. 282-92.

127. Alitalo, K., The lymphatic vasculature in disease. Nat Med, 2011. 17(11): p. 1371-80.

128. Sun, S.C. and J.T. Lie, Cardiac lymphatic obstruction: ultrastructure of acute-phase myocardial injury in dogs. Mayo Clin Proc, 1977. 52(12): p. 785-92.

129. Ullal, S.R., T.H. Kluge, and F. Gerbode, Functional and pathologic changes in the heart following chronic cardiac lymphatic obstruction. Surgery, 1972. 71(3): p. 328-34.

130. Szlavy, L., et al., Early disappearance of lymphatics draining ischemic myocardium in the dog. Angiology, 1987. 38(1 Pt 2): p. 73-84.

131. Taira, A., et al., Active drainage of cardiac lymph in relation to reduction in size of myocardial infarction: an experimental study. Angiology, 1990. 41(12): p. 1029-36.

132. Cui, Y., Impact of lymphatic vessels on the heart. Thorac Cardiovasc Surg, 2010. 58(1): p. 1-7.

133. Yotsumoto, G., et al., Experimental study of cardiac lymph dynamics and

edema formation in ischemia/reperfusion injury--with reference to the effect of hyaluronidase. Angiology, 1998. 49(4): p. 299-305.

134. Sutton, M.G. and N. Sharpe, Left ventricular remodeling after myocardial infarction: pathophysiology and therapy. Circulation, 2000. 101(25): p. 2981-8.

135. Brilla, C.G., J.S. Janicki, and K.T. Weber, Impaired diastolic function and coronary reserve in genetic hypertension. Role of interstitial fibrosis and medial thickening of intramyocardial coronary arteries. Circ Res, 1991. 69(1): p. 107-15.

136. Gramley, F., et al., Hypoxia and myocardial remodeling in human cardiac allografts: a time-course study. J Heart Lung Transplant, 2009. 28(11): p. 1119-26.

137. Laine, G.A. and S.J. Allen, Left ventricular myocardial edema. Lymph flow, interstitial fibrosis, and cardiac function. Circ Res, 1991. 68(6): p. 1713-21.

138. Casley-Smith, J.R. and J.R. Casley-Smith, The pathophysiology of lymphedema and the action of benzo-pyrones in reducing it. Lymphology, 1988. 21(3): p. 190-4.

139. Davis, K.L., et al., Effects of myocardial edema on the development of myocardial interstitial fibrosis. Microcirculation, 2000. 7(4): p. 269-80.

140. Westphal, C., et al., Effects of estrogen, an ERalpha agonist and raloxifene on pressure overload induced cardiac hypertrophy. PLoS One, 2012. 7(12): p. e50802.

Curriculum Vitae

Name	Xiang Zhang
Address for correspondence	Bonhoefferufer 14, 10589 Berlin Germany
	Tel: +49 178 1492076
	E-mail: xiang820312@gmail.com
Date and place of birth	12.03.1982 Hebei China
Nationality/ citizenship	China PR
Gender	Male

Primary and secondary Education:

07, 1989-07.2000   primary and secondary school in Shijiazhuang Hebei, China

Higher education:

09, 2000-06.2006 Bachelor qualification degree in Clinical medicine,

Harbin Medical University, China

09, 2006-06, 2009 Master qualification degree in Internal Medicine (Cardiology)

Harbin Medical University, China

05,2000-2014 Dr.med. studies

Medizinischen Fakultät Charité – Universitätsmedizin Berlin, Germany

Professional experience:

07, 2009- until now   Physician

Department of Cardiology the 4th Affiliated Hospital of Harbin Medical University, China

List of publications

Mahmoodzadeh S, Leber J, Zhang X, Jaisser F, Messaoudi S, et al. (2014) Cardiomyocyte-specific Estrogen Receptor Alpha Increases Angiogenesis, Lymphangiogenesis and Reduces Fibrosis in the Female Mouse Heart Post-Myocardial Infarction. J Cell Sci Ther 5:153. doi: 10.4172/2157-7013.1000153

http://dx.doi.org/10.4172/2157-7013.1000153

Acknowledgments/Danksagung

I would like to express my deep and sincere gratitude to my advisor professor Dr. Vera Regitz-Zagrosek and my supervisor Dr. Shokoufeh Mahmoodzadeh. I am grateful for their guidance and support and for providing me the opportunity to become a member of Prof. Regitz-Zagrosek's lab. I am so inspired by their passion for science, honesty in research and commitment to be a successful scientist.

Next, I need to thank all the people who create such a good atmosphere in the lab. Dr. Elke Dworatzek, Dr. George Petrov, Arne Kuehne.

I would also like to acknowledge all my committee members: Joachim Leber, Britta Fielitz, Vanessa Riese and Jenny Thomas, who spent countless hours in the lab explaining and showing me how to do everything and for sacrificing his time to help me.

I would like to thank all the past and present members of Prof. Regitz-Zagrosek's lab for their friendship and help and for their efforts and assistance.

Finally I want to thank my entire family for their unconditional love and support. Most of all, I want to thank my parents Lingjun Zhang, Hua Han, for everything they did for me. I also want to thank my friend Dietmar Naumann. Words can't express the love and gratitude I have for them. Their happiness and health are my biggest wish.

To each of the above, I extend my deepest appreciation

Berlin, 2014

List of abbreviations

BERKO, estrogen receptor beta knockout

BSA, bovine serum albumin

CAD, coronary artery disease

cDNA, complementary DNA

CM, cardiomyocyte

DAPI, 4'6'-diamidino-2-phenylindole dihydrochloride

DNA, deoxyribonucleic acid

E2, 17 β-estradiol

EC, endothelial cell

EDTA, ethylenediaminetetraacetic acid

ERα, estrogen receptor alpha

ERα-OE, cardiomyocyte-specific ERa overexpression

ERβ, estrogen receptor beta

ERKO, estrogen receptor alpha knock-out

ERs, estrogen receptors

H&E staining, hematoxylin and eosin staining

HIF, hypoxia inducible factor

IF, immunofluorescence

IHD, ischemic heart disease

I/R, ischemia-reperfusion

LAD left anterior descending coronary artery

LD, lymphatics density

LECs, lymphatic endothelial cells

LV, left ventricle

LVM, left ventricle mass

LYVE-1, lymphatic vessel endothelial hyaluronan receptor-1

MI, myocardial infarction

MMPs, matrix metalloproteinases

mRNA, messenger ribonucleic acid

PBS, phosphate buffered saline

PCR, polymerase Chain Reaction

PECAM-1/CD31, platelet endothelial cell adhesion molecule-1

RT-PCR, reverse transcription- polymerase chain reaction

SEM, standard error of the mean

TetR, tetracycline repressor

TIMPs, tissue inhibitors of metalloproteinases

TL, tibia length

TRE, tetracycline response element

ttA, tetracycline-controlled transactivator

VEGF, vascular endothelial growth factor

WT, wild type

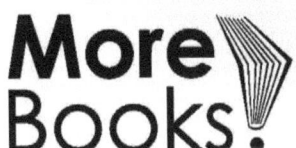
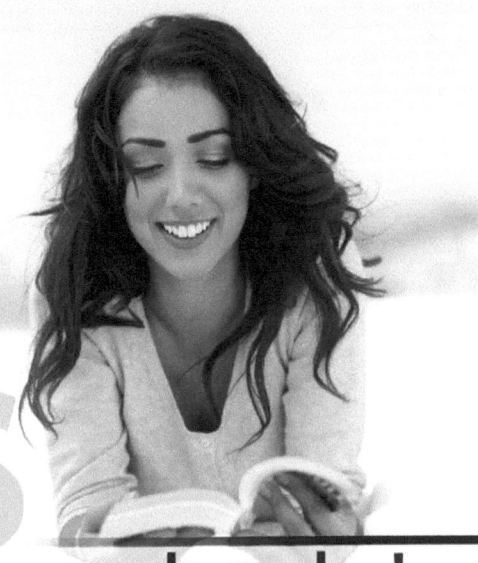

I want morebooks!

Buy your books fast and straightforward online - at one of the world's fastest growing online book stores! Environmentally sound due to Print-on-Demand technologies.

Buy your books online at
www.get-morebooks.com

Kaufen Sie Ihre Bücher schnell und unkompliziert online – auf einer der am schnellsten wachsenden Buchhandelsplattformen weltweit!
Dank Print-On-Demand umwelt- und ressourcenschonend produziert.

Bücher schneller online kaufen
www.morebooks.de

OmniScriptum Marketing DEU GmbH
Heinrich-Böcking-Str. 6-8
D - 66121 Saarbrücken
Telefax: +49 681 93 81 567-9

info@omniscriptum.com
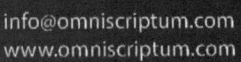
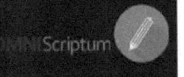

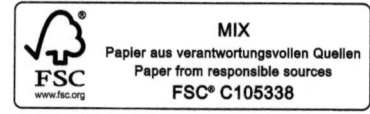

Printed by Books on Demand GmbH, Norderstedt / Germany